Exam Room
COMMUNICATION
for Veterinarians

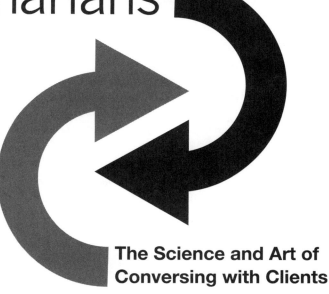

**The Science and Art of
Conversing with Clients**

Jon Klingborg, DVM, Distinguished Practitioner

AAHA
press

AAHA
press

American Animal Hospital Association Press
12575 West Bayaud Avenue
Lakewood, Colorado 80228 USA
303/986-2800 or 800/883-6301
press.aahanet.org

ISBN 978-1-58326-164-4

Library of Congress Cataloging-in-Publication Data

Klingborg, Jon.
  Exam room communication for veterinarians : the science and art of conversing with clients
    p. ; cm.
  Includes bibliographical references and index.
  ISBN 978-1-58326-164-4 (pbk. : alk. paper)
  I. American Animal Hospital Association. II. Title.
  [DNLM: 1. Communication. 2. Veterinary Medicine—methods. 3. Physical Examination—veterinary. 4. Professional-Patient Relations. 5. Veterinarians—psychology. SF 610.5]

  636.089—dc23
                        2011034546

Cover design by Erin Johnson Design
Interior design by Planet X Design

Printed in the United States of America
11 12 13 / 10 9 8 7 6 5 4 3 2 1

To the fabulous four-legged critters and their equally entertaining owners who make my veterinary career so worthwhile.

Contents

Preface   vii

Acknowledgments   ix

Part I. The Science of Veterinary Communication

Chapter 1.   Better Communication—What's in It for Me?   3

Chapter 2.   What Do Clients Really Want?   15

Chapter 3.   Verbal and Nonverbal Communication During the OFFICE Call   21

Chapter 4.   Grief Communication and Euthanasia   47

Part II. The Art of Conversing with Clients

Chapter 5.   Cognitive and Social Styles   57

Chapter 6.   Determining Cognitive Style   65

Chapter 7.   The Hawk   69

Chapter 8.   The Dog   79

Chapter 9.   The Kitten   89

Chapter 10.   The Owl   99

Chapter 11.   Conversing with All Cognitive Styles via the FALE System   111

Chapter 12.   Assessing Your Own Veterinary Conversation Style   117

Chapter 13.   Field Guide to Veterinary Personality Types   123

Chapter 14.   Avoiding Conversation Quicksand   145

Chapter 15.   Using Communication to Combat Burnout and Create Job Satisfaction   157

Appendix A: Personality Assessment   163

Appendix B: Burnout Inventory   167

Appendix C: Hobby Suggestions Based on Social-Cognitive Styles   169

References   171

Resources   181

Index   183

About the Author   195

Preface

This book is a practical guide to the most intriguing animal that veterinarians encounter on a daily basis, the human being. This is not intended as a lark. In fact, you will find that the thoroughly referenced information herein derives from copious literature regarding people's conversation styles and extensively draws on the science of medical communication.

To make it easy to navigate, material is divided into two parts. Part One, "The Science of Veterinary Communication," provides an overview of the tools you'll need to successfully communicate in the exam room. Part Two, "The Art of Conversing with Clients," presents a framework with which to understand all types of clients and to clarify their motivations, concerns, and driving forces.

As a veterinary practitioner preparing a book intended for his colleagues, I wanted to address a common challenge. Capable veterinarians learn to adapt a treatment plan to a particular animal's needs; however, many fail to adapt their communication style to meet the individual needs of their client. Why? Because no one has shown them how.

If you are a veterinarian and are seeking to improve your communication skills or understand your more challenging clients—well, congratulations! You have taken the next step to becoming a better doctor with more dedicated clients and greater job satisfaction.

Exam Room Communication for Veterinarians: The Science and Art of Conversing with Clients is precisely the book you need to take that next step toward practice excellence. Clients can be confusing and complicated. My hope is that you will come to consider this book as a Rosetta stone that aids in translating the curious language in which clients speak.

Acknowledgments

In spite of abundant wishful thinking, this book just wouldn't write itself. Instead, it exists because of some very important people.

I want to thank my parents, Don and Beverly, who inspire and guide me with their energy, intelligence, and love; my wife Kim, who is supportive, creative, and fun in equal measures; my sons Patrick and Aaron, who are wonderful in their own brilliant ways; and my stepdaughter Tina, who never doubted that I would get this book published.

A few truly excellent teachers have influenced and shaped me over the years. A special thanks to Mrs. Risley, first grade; Mr. Burns, fourth grade; Mrs. Werth, seventh grade; Mr. Burns and Mr. Ragonut, eighth grade; and in high school, Mr. Bell (biology), Mr. Rose (English), Mr. Withers (physics), and Frau Stein (German). You are appreciated and not forgotten.

Finally, I must thank AAHA for having, in my humble opinion, the courage and wisdom to publish this book. AAHA not only talks the talk about the importance of communication but also walks the walk. Thanks to my editor, Bess Maher, who improved every aspect of this book with her keen insight.

PART ONE

The Science of Veterinary Communication

Clients do us a favor when they choose our veterinary clinic over the competition. To retain these clients, we must be certain to address their needs.

Chapter 1 addresses the question, "Better communication—what's in it for me?" In answering this question, it explores the many reasons why improving our communication skills with clients improves the quality of our practice, reduces conflict, and increases job satisfaction and income.

By analyzing the question "What do clients really want?" Chapter 2 offers a look at the latest research on both veterinary clients and human patients to gain deeper understanding of pet owners' needs.

Chapter 3 takes a fresh look at the OFFICE call and discusses six important elements that go into each call. Verbal and nonverbal communication are discussed, as well as ways of assessing and improving one's likeability. This chapter also introduces the concept of the veterinarian as an advisor, rather than as an expert. The long-term benefits of an advisor-client relationship are substantial, but this dynamic differs from that more commonly seen in traditional paternal or authoritarian health care.

CHAPTER 1

Better Communication—What's in It for Me?

What's in it for you? Actually, that's a very good question. The payoffs for improved client communication are extensive and include the following:

- Reduced client conflict
- Reduced risk of lawsuit
- Greater client retention
- Growing client base
- Better compliance
- Increased compensation
- A more enjoyable work environment
- Greater career success

Reduced Client Conflict

Conflict in the exam room occurs for many reasons, but most difficult situations arise when veterinarians fail to recognize or address clients' needs.[1,2]

If a veterinarian doesn't address clients' concerns or provide the information they need, then conflict is going to result, especially if the veterinarian doesn't believe that clients' concerns are a high priority.

Over time in their practice, observant veterinarians start to recognize the unique traits of individual pet owners: Some owners want all of the details, and others just want to know that everything is going to be okay.[3] Conversations in nearly every exam room fall into one of two categories: wellness-oriented and problem-oriented. If clients voice a concern about their pet (no matter how minor it may seem to the doctor), then that concern must become a high priority, and the veterinarian should shift into problem-oriented mode to make certain client that needs are being met.

For example, a client may be more worried about his or her dog's bad breath than about the possibility that it might be in early congestive heart failure. However, if the veterinarian ignores the possible dental issue, then the client will be less receptive to discussing heart disease. As pointed out in *Verbal Judo: The Gentle Art of Persuasion,* "the first principle . . . is not to resist your [client]. Instead, move with him and redirect his energy. Ignoring or dismissing a question is the same as resisting it."[4(p43)]

Also remember the adage, "It's not what you say but how you say it." Easy enough, but most people learn this lesson the hard way—for example, by using the wrong tone of voice when speaking with someone. As you gain an understanding of a range of personality types and conversation styles, you'll become adept at tailoring your delivery of lab work and other information to individual clients and their need for a presentation that might be general, specific, theoretical, or practical. Answer their questions, and clients will know that you respect them and care about their pet.[5]

Reduced Risk of Lawsuit

Sure, some veterinarians are bad apples, but a significant number of formal client complaints actually stem from misunderstandings caused by poor communication.[*,6–10]

A veterinarian writing for the California licensing board summed it up in this way: "Many of the complaints received by the Veterinary Medical Board have very little to do with the actual care of the patient received. Some can be relegated to communication challenges."[11] Even in less litigious Canada, it was determined that "if practitioners are sued, . . . [the underlying reason] is more likely because of poor communication skills than medical or surgical ones." [†,12(p1),13]

Every practicing veterinarian knows that cases don't always work out the way you want or expect. Avoiding the complaint in the first place by communicating clearly is your best defense against a possible lawsuit or licensing board review.[14,15]

Greater Client Retention

The average dog owner spends an estimated $356 to $532 annually on medical care, and the average cat owner spends between $190 and $278.[16] With these numbers in mind, it's fair to ask, "How much money do you lose every time you lose a client?"

A *JAVMA* study determined that veterinarians who ranked in the top third in terms of client retention (the number of active clients retained over a period of time) had an individual annual income of $15,560 more than their bottom-third counterparts.[17,18] Veterinarians who ranked highly with regard to client loyalty (how likely it is a client will tolerate inconvenience to see his or her preferred veterinarian) had an individual annual income of $28,900 more than their bottom-third colleagues.[18] As for attracting new clients, this study revealed that new client development increased income by only $2,880 for the highest-scoring veterinarians. In other words, retaining a client will net you about three times more than the effort of finding new clients, and maintaining loyalty will net you 10 times more than a strong client development program.[18]

The Pareto principle states that 80 percent of income is derived from 20 percent of clients.[19,20] These regular customers are the ones that you need to retain—it's much more cost-effective to keep an established client coming in the door than to find a new client.

Every community seems to have one marginal veterinarian with great communication skills; if your veterinarian is like mine, he or she has such a loyal clientele that they are practically a fan club. Imagine how powerful it would be if you could create a fan club for your own practice by combining high-quality medicine and great communication skills.

Practice long enough and you will have ups and downs with the same client: an ear infection that didn't clear up with the first few treatments, an orthopedic case that took longer than expected to heal, a spay surgery site that became infected. Whether the client stays with you will be based on your ability to communicate with him or her.[21,22]

Growing Client Base

A 2004 *Wall Street Journal* survey asked the question, "What do you value in selecting your doctor?"[‡,23] Following is a list of the most important criteria selected by respondents (refer to Table 1.1 for complete results).

1. Treats you with dignity and respect (85 percent)
2. Listens carefully (84 percent)
3. Is easy to talk to (84 percent)
4. Truly cares about you and your health (81 percent)
5. Has good medical judgment (80 percent)
6. Asks you good questions and is easy to understand (79 percent)
7. Is up-to-date with the latest treatments (78 percent)

The *Wall Street Journal* survey underscored that, to most people, communication is more important than medical ability. Medical judgment was the fifth most important criterion; being up-to-date with the latest treatments was seventh. According to the responses, good communication clearly reigns supreme when choosing a doctor. Expressions of caring, clarity of communication, and how well the person was treated, listened to, and talked to were also very important.

TABLE 1.1 *Wall Street Journal (WSJ)* Survey Top Ten Results

Question A: Which of the following qualities are extremely important to you in the doctor or doctors who treat you?

Question B: Which of the following phrases, if any, do you think describe your current doctor well?	Extremely Important (%)	Describes Your Doctor Well (%)
Treats you with dignity and respect	85	73
Listens carefully to your health care concerns and questions	84	68
Is easy to talk to	84	69
Takes your concerns seriously	83	69
Is willing to spend enough time with you	81	62
Truly cares about you and your health	81	63
Has good medical judgment	80	65
Asks you good questions to really understand your medical conditions and your needs	79	54
Is up-to-date with the latest medical research and medical treatment	78	54
Can see you at short notice, if necessary	71	53

Methodology: This WSJ poll was conducted online in the U.S. between Sept. 21 and 23, 2004 among a nationwide cross section of 2,267 adults. Figures for age, sex, race/ethnicity, education, income and region were weighted where necessary to align with population proportions. Propensity score weighting was also used to adjust for respondents' propensity to be online. In theory, with probability samples of this size, one could say with 95% certainty that the results have a sampling error of ±3 percentage points of what they would be if the entire U.S. adult population had been polled with complete accuracy. This online sample was not a probability sample.

Of course, this survey concerned physicians, and most of the research available is also focused on MDs, not DVMs or VMDs. It doesn't take a great leap, however, to realize that these criteria are important on the veterinary side, too.[13,24]

As noted by Coe et al., both pet owners and veterinarians agreed that it is difficult for clients to accurately evaluate a veterinarian's competence, and although clients "trust that the veterinarian has the knowledge and skills," it was apparent that one of the ways veterinarians indirectly reinforce this belief is through the confidence with which they speak and their ability to communicate in terms a client can understand.[25(p1075)]

Historically, clients chose their veterinarian on the basis of several criteria, such as location, price, hours, word of mouth, and Yellow Pages advertising.[26,27] In the past decade, however, this has begun to change, with a 250 percent increase in owners who are selecting their veterinarian on the basis of a "personal recommendation."[27]

The 2009 *Veterinary Economics* magazine "State of the Industry" study showed that the most successful marketing method was a client referral program—a word-of-mouth tool by which existing clients get incentives for sending new clients to your door.[§,28] This program was three times more important than a Yellow Pages advertisement and seven times more important than a practice's website.

As social media such as Facebook, Twitter, and Yelp become standard agents for interactive dialogue and communication, veterinarians will find that clients select their services as a result of "word-of-mouth" online reviews. Seventy-four percent of respondents to one survey said they were influenced by the reviews they read on social media when purchasing a product, and another study showed that 73 percent of moms trust an online social community when looking for recommendations.[29,30]

The use of social media is still in its infancy, but linking with clients through Internet sites will certainly become an important means of future marketing for veterinarians. One study showed that those who "like" a restaurant's Facebook page visited the chain 20 percent more frequently and spent 33 percent more money.[§,31] A *Forbes* report from 2010 showed that people who "liked" a company's Facebook page were 41 percent more likely to recommend that company and 28 percent more likely to continue using it.[32] Imagine if you could get people to "like" your veterinary clinic and then send or link to online endorsements to encourage their friends to come see you!

The next generation of clients is going to find a new veterinarian through an Internet search engine, read online reviews of that veterinary clinic, and then print out a map and drive to the highest-rated facility. If you have a strong, positive Internet presence, your clinic will continue to flourish.[33] Positive word of mouth via online reviews will be created by excellent communication and good medical outcomes. On the flip side, poor interpersonal skills will be blogged about, tweeted about, and similarly broadcast in this age of the Internet.

Better Compliance

For years, veterinary journals have talked about poor client compliance.[34–37] The prevailing sentiment has been that veterinarians are unlikely to improve client compliance because clients do a very poor job of complying in general, even when it is for their personal health.[38]

In 2003, an American Animal Hospital Association (AAHA) study revealed that 60 percent of clients felt that veterinarians didn't make it clear how important their health care recommendations really were to the pet's well-being.[39] At the same time, 60 percent of veterinarians said poor compliance was the client's fault.

Over the next four years, AAHA worked with its member hospitals and created a formula for dealing with the problem, called *CRAFT*: Compliance = Recommendation + Acceptance + Follow Through. The follow-up 2008 study showed an improvement in client compliance ranging from 64 to 73 percent across all parameters.[40]

A commitment to improved communication increased client compliance.

The overarching focus of CRAFT was increasing the communication with the client, and the results were clear that a commitment to improved communication increased client compliance. In 2010, *Veterinary Economics* detailed one hospital's 17 percent increase in diagnostic bloodwork within two years of establishing protocols that communicated the lab work's importance.[**,41]

The reality is that veterinarians fall short when it comes to completely engaging clients when recommending treatment or diagnostic protocols. The book *Leveraging Your Communication Style* suggests appealing to "three points of engagement," that is, speaking to the head, heart, and feet.[42(p5)] Veterinarians are good at appealing to the head (intellectual need for tests) and the heart (attachment to the animal), but they can fail to compel the feet into action by asking the client to agree to a recommended service.

In sales jargon, appealing to the feet is called *closing the deal*. The truth is that clients don't always recognize when veterinarians have made a recommendation for action, and "a stealth recommendation is useless to your patients, your clients, and your practice."[43]

The crux of the issue is that to gain client acceptance, veterinarians must sell the service—and even the most stoic veterinarian can become squeamish when talking about money. Veterinarians hesitate to talk about money and sell services for several reasons:[44]

- Society often equates the size of the wallet with personal worth and value, making frank money discussions the last taboo in U.S. culture.
- Doctors feel that discussing the cost of services conflicts with their role as healers. Will clients think that tests are being recommended simply because the doctor will financially gain?[45] After all, veterinarians want to celebrate the human-animal bond, not market it.[46]
- In a busy clinical setting, the time a doctor uses to discuss money issues will take away from time spent doing other important tasks, such as treating other patients and talking with owners about their pet's well-being.[47]
- Many veterinarians have no idea how their practice's fee schedule was created and what the actual costs (facility, materials, staff, time) of any service really are.[48]

To successfully engage clients in "money talk," veterinarians should discuss the benefits of a certain course of action. By recognizing and addressing the cost:benefit ratio (from the client's perspective), veterinarians can market their services without feeling like used-car salespeople. This approach also creates a better dynamic with the client, who becomes less focused on what service you are selling than on why it is needed.

Increased Compensation

AAHA's 2003 study on compliance gaps estimated that individual veterinarians lost about $650,000 in revenue opportunities every year.[39] If you're a practice owner, that's a substantial loss of business income; if you're an associate veterinarian paid at 20 percent, that means your yearly paycheck could have been $100,000 larger.

Some practitioners feel that it's tacky or inappropriate to discuss methods of increasing compensation, yet this isn't a conversation for mercenaries alone. Aside from the personal benefits of increasing income, the reality is that a profitable practice is good for patients; after all, net income is what allows veterinarians to buy new equipment, keep the clinic looking clean and professional, and retain a quality staff.

Communication is a key driver in increasing income—it has a direct influence on the number of clients seen and the average transaction fee. As pointed out in *Communicating with Today's Patient*, "to have a successful practice any clinician must have three core competencies: the science, the art, and the business of medicine."[49] Communication is a cornerstone of the art and business of veterinary medicine.

More Enjoyable Work Environment

It shouldn't be a big leap to realize that all the rewards of better communication are intertwined—if you're communicating better and your clients are happier, then conflict will be reduced and the work environment will be more enjoyable.

> *Every doctor in the practice, even the new associate, has some responsibility for creating, fostering, and communicating a culture of quality care and client satisfaction.*

When one looks at the reasons why a clinic team has become dysfunctional, the importance of communication is clear. Everything from errors in treatment to failure to work as a group has a foundation in poor communication.[50] Having an effective and efficient team requires not only that the right people be in the right places, but also that they be unified by a common purpose—what may be best referred to as a *culture*. This culture is united in a mission to help animals through quality care and regards the client as an opportunity rather than an obstacle. Every doctor in the practice, even the new associate, has some responsibility for creating, fostering, and communicating a culture of quality care and client satisfaction.

When the team is united as part of the same culture, petty conflicts fade into the background and the work environment is much more enjoyable for all. Clients certainly perceive this positive energy, and it bonds them to your practice even more.

Greater Career Success

Research has identified six essentials that define career success as a veterinarian:[51]

1. Fulfillment from work
2. Balancing relationships
3. Pursuing personal goals
4. Helping others
5. Making enough money
6. Participating in the profession

Most of these essentials of career success clearly have good communication as a common thread. Research has shown that professional satisfaction leads to better communication that results in even greater satisfaction.[††,49] Better interpersonal rapport, personal warmth, and affection toward clients also increase professional satisfaction.[‡‡,52]

Notes

[*]"The existence of disciplinary policies and procedures serves as a balance between the emotions and desires of the pet owner and the standards and practices of the veterinarian.

[†]The extra cost of malpractice lawsuits is a proportion of health spending in both the United States (0.46

percent) and Canada (0.27 percent). In Canada, the total cost of settlements, legal fees, and insurance comes to $4 per person each year, but in the United States, it's $16. Malpractice suits are far more common in the United States, with 350 percent more suits filed each year per person.[12]

‡This poll was conducted online in the United States from September 21 to 23, 2004, among a nationwide cross section of 2,267 adults.

¶This study asked, "What marketing method results in the most customers?" Among the responses were client referral program, 48 percent; Yellow Pages, 15 percent; and practice website, 7 percent.

§A restaurant called Dessert Gallery in Houston, Texas, asked 700 clients to become fans; 75 did. Those who did visited the chain 20 percent more frequently than those who didn't and spent 33 percent more overall and were emotionally more attached, but only 5 percent of clients became fans.

**Bells Ferry Veterinary Hospital in Acworth, Georgia, reported a 17 percent increase in diagnostic bloodwork within two years of establishing and communicating protocols for diagnostic lab work.

††"Your professional satisfaction is still affected by your day-to-day communications with patients; conversely, your communications with patients are profoundly influenced by your degree of professional satisfaction."[49(p238)]

‡‡"The positive regard associated with patient satisfaction with care and judgments of good performance, interpersonal rapport, and personal warmth and affection, are all likely to inspire physician satisfaction."[52(p144)]

CHAPTER 2

What Do Clients Really Want?

Top Three Client Needs

Focus group studies have helped shed some light on what clients really want from their experience at your clinic. These needs fall under three main themes:[1,5,25,49,52–54]

1. Clients want you to respect them and the relationship they've chosen with their pet.

2. Clients want to understand their pet's problem and have you resolve it.

3. Clients want to feel positive about their experience at your clinic.

Clients Want You to Respect Them and the Relationship They've Chosen with Their Pet

Every client's relationship with his or her pet is unique. Some owners see their pets as "employees" that are expected to work herding livestock or acting as sentries; others see their pets as best friends or nurturers, as children, or even as soul mates.[55] It's important to remember that there isn't one right way to be a pet owner.

As noted in a 2004 *Wall Street Journal* poll (see Chapter 1 and Table 1.1), respondents rated being treated with dignity and respect as the most important criterion when evaluating a doctor.[23]

In the veterinary realm, respect comes in many forms, including not keeping clients waiting too long, using the owner's and pet's names, working as an advisor instead of taking a more authoritarian approach, providing owners with a range of options, and allowing them to decide for themselves what they can or will do for their pets.[1,5,22,25,53]

Good Owners Behaving Badly

When potentially good clients have neglected a pet, it is seldom beneficial to berate them for making a bad choice or no choice (inactivity) for the animal. Many bad owners are simply misinformed or are following some family tradition of pet care—what has been modeled to them during their upbringing. If you respect these owners and educate them, you'll have great clients for the life of the pet; just as important, you'll have an opportunity to improve the culture of pet care in that person's community. However, if you browbeat clients for making bad decisions about their pet, they may realize that they have been negligent but also "shoot the messenger" and consider choosing you for a veterinarian as their biggest mistake. Of course, I'm not suggesting you turn a blind eye to animal cruelty or neglect, but "bad" owners can be engaged in a constructive fashion that helps them understand the error of their ways.

Clients Want to Understand Their Pet's Problem and Have You Resolve It

The theme of "wanting to understand the doctor" has appeared in numerous studies and surveys.[1,5,25,56-58] After all those years of college, you'd think veterinarians would've learned that people don't all speak or think the way they do. Unfortunately, it comes as a surprise to many practitioners that they've failed to communicate with their clients, leaving owners either to conclude that "the doctor must be smart because I didn't understand him" or to worry they'll "look even more stupid" if they ask the doctor for clarification. Unfortunately, some clients are simply too intimidated to ask questions. In Part Two of this book, you'll learn to identify personality types of clients who may have questions but are too afraid to ask them.

Moreover, if staff are being bombarded with a client's questions after the exam, the problem may not be with the client but with the client's exam room experience. In other words, the doctor's demeanor or explanation was lacking in some way.

It's a common mistake to think that clients are paying for a veterinarian's time and knowledge. True, you are spending valuable time with clients, but they are also giving up their time to be with you, so the concept of time being bought and sold doesn't really make sense. After all, whose time is more valuable? (Large-animal practitioners who bill by the hour

The commodities that veterinarians sell are useful information and technical expertise.

should realize that hourly billing is done not because their knowledge flows at a steady hourly rate, but because it improves client efficiency.)

When it comes to paying for veterinarians' storehouse of knowledge, the reality is that clients have no means of determining what a doctor knows or doesn't know—there just isn't a reliable tool to measure knowledge. In actuality, the commodities that veterinarians sell are useful information and technical expertise. It's key to realize that clients define what is considered useful information—it's what's important to them.

The following list outlines how, when surveyed, veterinary clients wanted information:[25]

- **Explained:** Owners wanted to understand their pet's problem, diagnosis, treatment, and alternative therapies.
- **Presented up front:** Owners desired a candid accounting of both the good and the bad aspects of a diagnosis or treatment plan.

- **Available in various forms:** Veterinary clients wanted access to print and Internet materials that would allow them to gain a deeper understanding of their pet's problem outside the exam room.

When clients leave without useful information in hand or in mind, they haven't really gotten their money's worth.

Congenial, not Congenital

Clients actually prefer that their doctor speak using "real" words—the kind of words that clients might use in everyday (polite) conversation.[23,57,59] Veterinarians and physicians both seem to worry that using real words makes them seem less intelligent to the client, but the opposite is actually true.[60–62] A classic example is the veterinarian's use of the word *congenital*. Although it may be common in the vernacular of the veterinary profession, I'm certain that some clients, when they see a word including *genital*, aren't thinking about birth defects or genetic problems. My favorite example of a misunderstanding relates to a foreleg amputation in a pet. The horrified owner thought the discussion was about a "four-leg" amputation and couldn't understand how the poor animal was ever going to walk again.

The reality is that successful communication is defined as that in which information is accurately transferred from one person to another. Referring to an upset stomach as gastroenteritis may make you sound smart, but it does nothing to increase the client's understanding.

What's the Problem?

In the spirit of "the customer is always right," veterinarians should recite the mantra "If it's a problem

---

Overcoming the Language Barrier

It's actually fun and rewarding to speak real English in the exam room!

- "Cardiomyopathy" becomes "weakened heart muscle."
- "Hip dysplasia" is now "a poor fit between the ball and socket of the hip."
- A "corneal abrasion" is explained as "a wound of the eye, like when you fell down as a kid and skinned your knee. It was big and it hurt a lot, but wasn't very deep."

Clients will love you for speaking their language, and it doesn't diminish your knowledge one bit.

for the client, then it's a problem for me, too." Veterinarians learn early to develop and prioritize a problem list. This organizational tool is critical to the science of healing. As veterinarians move through the physical exam, new problems may emerge and change the ranking of older problems. Unfortunately, many veterinarians seem to regard themselves as "keepers of the problem list" and try to impose their priorities on the owner.[53]

What if the client is more worried about the dog's cough keeping him or her awake at night than that the cough might be caused by heart disease? If the client's primary complaint isn't addressed, then he or she is unlikely to buy in to the expensive diagnostic or treatment plan just because the doctor thinks the other problem is more important. This doesn't mean a veterinarian should ignore heart disease and prescribe cough medicine just to keep the client happy; the client should be satisfied with an explanation of how the cough and the heart disease are interrelated. The client will become fully engaged when the doctor has explained how the presence (or absence) of a cough can be used to measure the progression of the pet's heart disease.

> *"If it's a problem for the client, then it's a problem for me, too."*

Clients Want to Feel Positive About Their Experience at Your Clinic

If clients are going to return to your hospital, they need to feel positive about the experience. *Feeling positive* is different from *feeling good*. Even a euthanasia appointment can be a positive experience if the owner feels that you were compassionate toward the animal and empathetic with him or her.

Clients are consumers, and consumers have choices. Clients in your clinic have done you a favor by spending their money at your facility. Ultimately, they want to trust you as well, but trust takes time. Psychologists will tell you that people don't trust people they don't like, and people don't like people who don't seem to like them. We'll discuss increasing your likeability in the next chapter, but the concept is important enough to introduce now.

Research has shown that clients expect their veterinarians to listen to them and to ask the right questions.[25] What is interesting is that people can't seem to identify ahead of time how much listening or question-asking is appropriate, but they certainly recognize when they haven't had enough of either after an office call.

Conclusion

Clients' expectations are very clear. They want you to respect them and the relationship they've chosen with their pet; they want to understand what is wrong with their pet and resolve it, and to feel positive about their experience at your clinic. You can show clients respect in many ways, including being on time for the appointment, dressing appropriately, seeking to advise rather than lecture them, and addressing them by name.

Clients want to understand, and understanding comes from speaking a common language; using handouts, models, a dry-erase board, or other aids; explaining the problem and the options; and presenting the information all at once instead of holding something back.

Positive feelings are generated when clients think you respect and like them, when you speak in an understandable way, and when you listen and care enough to ask the right questions.

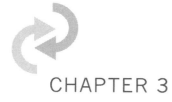

CHAPTER 3

Verbal and Nonverbal Communication During the OFFICE Call

Communication is typically divided into two main components: verbal and nonverbal. Simply stated, *verbal communication* is all about what is said out loud and focuses on the what and how of information that is shared, including not just the words but also the tone, warmth, and use of silence. *Nonverbal communication* consists of all the other stuff: body language, physical distance, gestures, facial expressions, and so on.

Separating verbal and nonverbal communication is traditional when discussing communication; however, this division is artificial, because in the exam room setting (and the rest of the world) both forms of communication occur at the same time. A veterinarian may say the right words but send a conflicting nonverbal message. For example, if you ask the client whether he or she has any more questions as you gather the chart and stethoscope, you're signaling that the time for questions is actually over. Verbal and nonverbal actions must send the same message for the client to feel at ease.

The OFFICE Call

Typically, the OFFICE call is divided into six sections: (1) O, outside the exam room; (2) F, first impression; (3) F, friendly talk; (4) I, inquiry; (5) C, communicate your findings; and (6) E, enlist the client and empathize.

Outside the Exam Room

Physical Preparation

Meeting client expectations includes how you look as well as how you act. An overwhelming 76 percent of clients want their doctor to wear a white lab coat.[63,64] Only 4.7 percent felt that casual attire was appropriate, which is an extremely low number—particularly when you realize that fewer than 6 percent of Americans don't believe astronauts actually landed on the moon.[65] In addition, clients thought scrubs were only slightly better than casual dress or a business suit (see Figure 3.1).

Why do clients want you to wear a white lab coat? Because the lab coat is the uniform of those who represent the science of healing. Your lab coat is a symbol that separates you from the quacks, shamans, and snake oil salespeople of the world.[66]

FIGURE 3.1 Client Preference for Doctor Dress[63,66]

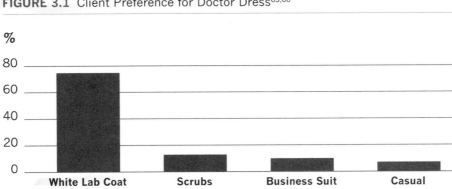

Veterinarians who reject dress codes often respond, "Judge me by what I know, not how I dress." Well, the fundamental problem with that response is that clients don't know what you know—after all, they didn't go to veterinary school. Therefore, a client's assessment of your abilities may be more superficial than you would like.

Multiple studies have shown that when a doctor wears a white lab coat, the client is more likely to do the following:[49,66-68]

- Trust the doctor.
- Believe the doctor is competent.
- View the doctor as meticulous and serious.
- Share private information.

Research has shown that two other tools of the trade give you credibility and should also be part of your uniform: a name badge and a stethoscope.[66,67]

The last part of your physical preparation is common sense: Make certain you don't appear to be in disarray. Your hair should be neat; shirt, buttoned; and lab coat, free of hair, bloodstains, and any other body fluids that veterinarians encounter on a daily basis.

Mental Preparation

Read the file. There really is no excuse for not having a basic idea why the client is in the exam room. Before entering, you should take a moment to familiarize yourself with the patient's and client's names. If another animal is in the exam room, ask your staff to alert you, so that you can say "hi" to him or her, too.

Likeability: A Great Sixth Impression

A client's impression of your practice (1) begins on the phone when the appointment is scheduled, (2) continues as the client turns into the parking lot, (3) is enhanced or diminished by the receptionists at the front desk, (4) is influenced by other people in the waiting room, and (5) is affected by the veterinary assistant who took the pet's initial history.

By the time you've entered the exam room, you may be the sixth nail in the coffin. This may be the one and only time you'll see these clients—or you may have an opportunity to win them over if you can wow them into forgiving any prior transgressions.

Unfortunately, good impressions are based on more than your knowledge or ability to diagnose the pet's problem. Whether it's fair or not, a good sixth impression is essentially a function of your *likeability*, the intangible quality that makes another person think, "I like you and want to listen to you."

In his book *The Likeability Factor: How to Boost Your L-Factor and Achieve Your Life's Dreams*, Tim Sanders stated:

> *The quality of your life and the strength of your relationships are the product of a choice—but not necessarily your choice. . . . Many of the determiners in your life are the choices that other people make. The more likeable you are, the more likely you are to be on the receiving end of positive choice, from which you benefit.*[69(p33)]

According to Pam Holloway's "Seven Components of Likeability," those who develop these seven components will increase their Likeability Quotient and have clients flocking to them:[70]

1. **Positive mental attitude.** Likeable people are able to make lemonade out of lemons. They find the positive spin on a negative situation and work to improve the problem at hand.

2. **Nonjudgmental nature.** Truly likeable people don't make obvious value judgments about others. They understand that every person is different and is often doing the best that he or she can, or if the person is truly difficult, they recognize that outside influences must be making him or her that way.

3. **Openness.** Likeable people are open to new ideas, new people, and new experiences and are willing to explore the alternatives.

4. **Secure.** Likeable people know who the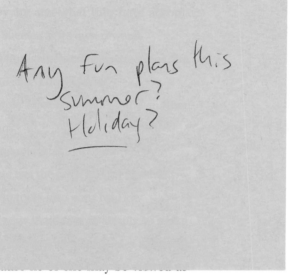
   plished and don't need to brag about it.

5. **Vulnerability.** Likeable people admit th
   sincerely self-deprecating, and are able

6. **See the other's perspective.** Likeable pe
   person's needs, obstacles, and motivatic

7. **People who like us.** People tend to like

Some folks are innately likeable, but everyo

with time and self-examination, you can put the

If you are shy, the first step to increasing

a commitment to do just that. In the precedin

reserved person may have an uphill battle, bec

lacking openness or security and may even be interpreted as being judgmental or

having a negative attitude. Use the "Likeability Assessment" in Figure 3.2 to help

determine how likeable you are.

The easiest way to seem more likeable is to try to find common interests with

your clients, for example a shared love of a particular breed or hobby. If a client car-

ries a book into the exam room, ask him or her about it: "Is that a good author? What

kind of books does she write?" Although it's more appropriate to do this after the pet's

issues have been addressed, it may help the exam to end on a "likeable" note.

All people want to be liked, and research has shown that people find doctors

who seem to like them to be more competent and caring.[71,72] Increased likeability

reduces stress and burnout for doctors; studies have confirmed that doctors who

are liked by their patients tend to have higher levels of job satisfaction.[73] As the

Beatles sang, "The love you take is equal to the love you make."[74]

It's Showtime

No one wants his or her doctor to be in a hurry. Before you walk into the exam room,

take a deep breath and cultivate a nonanxious presence.[75-77] Your clients have just

FIGURE 3.2 Likeability Assessment

Circle the answer in each pair of questions that describes you most of the time:

  a. I am good at reading people and usually an excellent judge of character.
  b. Some people really surprise or disappoint me—maybe I'm not as good at reading people as I thought.

  1. At a social gathering, I'd rather not talk about someone's hobbies, past jobs, and so on. Instead, let's find something that interests both of us and talk about that.
  2. I can talk to just about anyone at any time about their interests—hobbies, past jobs, accomplishments, and so forth.

  a. People see me as relaxed and easy to get along with.
  b. People don't always read me correctly and often seem to think that I'm tense or unhappy.

  1. Life is good, but I always want more.
  2. I smile often.

  a. I always try to find the positive in any situation and generally think that things will work out.
  b. I'm a realist—things don't always work out and I know that.

  1. There are still many things that I need or want, and I worry about missing those opportunities.
  2. I am generally happy and content with life.

  a. When talking with someone, most of the time I'd rather listen than talk about myself.
  b. The best conversation is when I can share many of my thoughts, feelings, and interests with others.

  1. At work, I'd rather do things by myself—it gets done right the first time and more quickly.
  2. My coworkers might consider me a good coach or a teacher. I try to build others' self-confidence.

  a. I make an effort to be patient with people.
  b. I tend to get frustrated or irritated with people quickly or on a regular basis.

  1. I don't like to be dependent on others and don't encourage them to be dependent on me.
  2. When my friends have a problem, they often seek me out to listen and advise them.

Scoring: Give yourself one point for each answer "a" or "2."
9–10 points: You aren't just likeable, you're the life of the party! Take care, though, that you're still able to draw boundaries so that clients don't take advantage of you as their new best friend.

7–8 points: You have high likeability, and clients will tell others about your excellent "pet-side" manner.

5–6 points: You need to improve your likeability if you hope to retain clients and grow your practice.

0–4 points: Your medical skills had better be darned good and your business sense savvy, because low likeability will drive clients away from your door. Don't worry, though; likeability can be improved.

hmmm – the "nonfacts" as an efficiency?

navigated a full parking lot, heard a chorus of rin commotion of a busy waiting room. So they are alre you might be too busy for their pet or their questio also more likely to think that you rushed through something.

On busy days, veterinarians tend to skip the mo (e.g., "How is Fluffy doing?") and get straight to the b to save time (e.g., "Is Fluffy eating?"). Surprisingly, stud ians who ask a number of lifestyle or social questions instead of focusing only on biomedical problems actually spend less time in the exam room.[78–80]

actually spend less time in the exam room.

So, asking more general questions about the patient can actually give you information more quickly than asking specific questions. You may also seem more relaxed and more willing to listen, so clients won't perceive that you're too busy for them.

First Impression

As you enter the exam room, introduce yourself or say "hi" to a regular client with direct eye contact, a smile, and an outstretched hand.[81] Entering the exam room with positive energy can change the mood. Presenting a calm and outgoing nature will soften the edge for the client who has been waiting longer than expected.[82]

Dr. Nalini Ambady, a Harvard professor of social psychology, has found that within 10 to 30 seconds of meeting someone, an individual has developed an impression of that person's competence, confidence, and enthusiasm.[83] This finding has major implications for veterinarians who are meeting a client for the first time and for maintaining an established client's trust.

Similar studies of student-teacher interaction have shown a positive correlation between a teacher's smile on first meeting a class and the overall evaluation of

---

Within 10 to 30 seconds of meeting someone, an individual has developed an impression of that person's competence, confidence, and enthusiasm.

---

that teacher at the end of the semester.[84,85] This positive response was seen in smiles as brief as two seconds or as long as 10 seconds.[85] In other words, an indelible positive impression can be generated in as little as two seconds! Think about your body language the next time you enter an exam room.

Although a smile goes a long way toward improving client satisfaction, if the client was kept waiting past the scheduled appointment time it is important to apologize as soon as you enter the exam room.[82,86] In most cases a simple sincere statement can defuse the tension. Perhaps say, "I apologize for your long wait," or offer an apology with an explanation such as "I'm sorry for your long wait; it is extremely busy today." Most clients will accept your apology and move on. Explain to clients who are still clearly angry that you will give their pet all the time it needs. If they're still angry by the end of the visit, then something else is probably bothering them.

You Should've Been in Pictures!

Enlist a staff member to videotape you during an office call.

Ask clients whether it's okay before the camera enters the room and explain that you're trying to put together a video about discussing health problems in pets. Assure them that the camera will be focused on you or their pet, so they don't need to be self-conscious.[78,97]

Assess your own performance in three ways:

1. **Watch the video as filmed.** Write down the positives and negatives.

2. **Turn off the sound and watch the video.** What mood does your facial expression or overall body language convey? Is it what you were trying to project? Write down the positives and negatives.

3. **Listen to the audio without looking at the video.** What do your vocal tones say? Are you speaking with dominance or warmth? Write down the positives and negatives.

This is a self-critique and is meant to be a learning experience. No one but you has to ever look at the video.

Friendly Talk

Numerous models of medical communication concern the importance of small talk, but few prioritize it as a key component of the exam room process.[87,88] It's ironic, because the two to three minutes spent creating rapport with clients has been shown to greatly increase client satisfaction and reduce the doctor's liability.[75,89]

A veterinarian who is willing to take time to engage in more casual exam room conversation sends several messages:[44]

- I have time for you and your pet.
- Our veterinarian-client relationship is more important than the business of one exam room transaction.
- I see you as an individual and not as something on an assembly line.

When you're engaged in friendly talk, it's difficult to come across as dominating, accusatory, or negative. Tone can be as important as the words people use, so friendly talk conveys warmth and caring, plus it increases levels of trust.[90–92]

On the basis of vocal tones in 20-second audio clips of surgeons talking with patients, one researcher was able to predict which surgeons would be sued and which wouldn't. She measured vocal tones that conveyed "dominance" versus "warmth" and found that those who displayed high dominance and low warmth were 2.7 times more likely to consult their attorney.[93] In other studies, patients were less satisfied with their care when the doctor asked specific, yes-or-no questions.[78,80,94,95]

However, too much social conversation can decrease the amount of information being shared, so doctors need to discipline themselves to shift from friendly talk to inquiry and stay on task.[96]

Inquiry

Find Out Why They're There

"What do you know? What do I know about what you know?" Share with clients what you understand about their pet's problem (from notations in the file and what the exam room technician has told you). Often, clients modify the problem or history that they gave the technician—perhaps they've had a bit more time to think about the situation and get it straight in their mind. This dialogue thus sets the stage for clients to share their problem list with you. As mentioned before, it is important to be mindful of what prompted clients to bring their pet to the clinic.[80]

"Where Does It Hurt?"

Ideally, you should initially ask more general open-ended questions—they tend to yield a broader type and depth of information and, to the client, feel a lot more like an inquiry and a lot less like an inquisition.[98,99]

Unfortunately, veterinarians don't spend much time either gathering information or asking open-ended questions. Research has shown that the inquiry phase of a typical veterinary visit makes up only 9 percent of the total conversation.[79] Moreover, the ratio of closed-ended to open-ended questions was 13:2. In other words, on average only about 13 percent of questions were open-ended. In 25 percent of the exams studied, the veterinarian did not ask any open-ended questions during the inquiry phase.[100]

The overwhelming use of closed-ended questions is the veterinary medical equivalent of going straight to exploratory surgery every time a pet is vomiting. Think of open-ended questions as the broad-spectrum tests (e.g., a blood panel) that give you a lot of general information, and of closed-ended questions as the specific tests (e.g., heartworm, blood urea nitrogen) that home in on a particular problem.

Starting with broad questions enables you to gather a breadth of information that may significantly alter your perception and understanding of the pet's problems. Not only is this inquiry style more satisfying, but it also builds rapport with clients,[100] because you are having a conversation with them, not cross-examining them.

Physical Exam

It's important that you perform a reasonably thorough exam every time you see a patient. Clients are paying for an exam, not just to have their pet's ears scoped. They may try to speed the process along and ask you to look at the pet's ears as soon as you've walked into the room. The best response is to explain that you're going to look the pet over from nose to tail to make sure you don't miss anything. Clients aren't likely to be upset because you're being more thorough, and they're also less likely to complain later because you didn't even look at "X."

Communicating the Plan: Are You the Expert or the Advisor?

As you begin to discuss your findings and explore the diagnostic and treatment options, you have a choice to make in terms of how you deliver the information. Do you speak to the client as though you were the expert or the advisor? According to David Maister, a former professor at Harvard Business School, 80 percent of clients "would prefer to hire a true advisor and, if they could find someone skilled in taking that approach, would be willing to pay a premium for it."[101]

> *Eighty percent of clients "would prefer to hire a true advisor and, if they could find someone skilled in taking that approach, would be willing to pay a premium for it."*

Of course, veterinarians are highly trained experts and advisors—the question here is one of style. Both styles have their appeal, although one probably suits your personality better than the other does. Experts and advisors serve different roles: Experts typically are hired by clients to solve a specific problem and are then dismissed—the relationship exists from one transaction to another and is not ongoing. Experts are usually sought out for their technical skills (ability to get the job done), but clients tend to be very concerned about getting their money's worth.

Advisors invest more in long-term relationships and are less interested in having things done their way every time. The advisor-client dynamic is more flexible than the expert-client dynamic because it gives clients more options and more responsibility in making decisions. In other words, although advisors may also be experts, in an advisor-client dynamic the advisor is an *expert guide*.

Many veterinarians (and other health professionals) would rather have an expert-client relationship because it allows them to take charge, is less emotionally draining, and has clearer boundaries—once the transaction is completed, the relationship is over. The disadvantage of expert-client interactions is that clients are much more likely to engage in negotiating and bargaining with the doctor.

The practical advantage to being an advisor is that loyal clients will spend more dollars in your veterinary clinic every year.

As with other experts whom the client might hire, such as a plumber or contractor, veterinarians are essentially bidding to perform their services. This potentially creates an adversarial situation in the exam room.

The advisor-client dynamic has some significant advantages. Advising is an interactive and ongoing process, which tends to create loyalty as clients see that your role is to help them.[*,101–103] It fosters a feeling of trust, and one of the main goals set by both parties is to preserve the relationship for the future. The practical advantage to being an advisor is that loyal clients will spend more dollars in your veterinary clinic every year.

The disadvantage of the advisor-client dynamic is that veterinarians must be willing to allow clients to make decisions in their own time frame, which may mean, for example, that clients decide to wait on a veterinarian-recommended hospitalized treatment and opt instead to try a course of medication at home. Of course, clients are always the ultimate decision makers. After all, it's their pocketbook and their pet. Another disadvantage is that, when compared with the role of an expert, the advisor role requires greater emotional and interpersonal commitment from veterinarians to engage and guide their clients. (See Table 3.1.)

TABLE 3.1 Expert or Advisor—Which Is Best?

Exam Room Behavior	Expert	Advisor
Relationship duration	Short term or transitional	Long-term
Feelings	"Buyer beware" atmosphere	Trust atmosphere
Strategy	Negotiate and bargain	Give options and provide guidance
Control	The expert knows what's right and does it	Client retains control and makes decisions
Focus	Getting the job done	Focus on the future
Emphasis	Technical skills	Interpersonal skills
Personality	Impersonal, detached	Personal, engaged
Listening style	Listen to what they're saying	Listen to what they're feeling and why they're feeling it
Communication style	Defensive, protective	Open, inquisitive
Main goal	Do it my way	Preserve the relationship
Commitment or loyalty	Until the job is done	Ongoing

Adapted and modified from Maister.[101]

Advisor in the Exam Room

As an advisor, you've agreed to a partnership with your clients; this means that you are there to help instead of harp. A key component of exam room communication is message delivery, and you must deliver the message—that is, information—in an understandable and agreeable way.

Keep in mind that whenever a veterinarian suggests that clients change their behavior, there is an implied criticism that what they're currently doing is not good enough. Whether the suggestion is to feed an overweight pet less food or to use a different flea product, it may put clients on the defensive. "The secret to success in conversation is to disagree without being disagreeable."[†] Never is this more true than in the exam room setting.

> *Keep in mind that whenever a veterinarian suggests that clients change their behavior, there is an implied criticism that what they're currently doing is not good enough.*

Think about how you would deliver advice if the client were one of your parents. The goal with clients or parents is the same: to help them to understand the situation as you see it and allow them to come to their own decision about the right course of action. Thus, rather than telling clients what to do, it is best to give them the pros and cons of several courses of action and then ask them for input. Of course, the veterinarian as an advisor hasn't given up responsibility for the case—he or she needs to consider and present the best options for the pet on the basis of his or her professional experience and medical intuition.

In the case of a chronic ear infection, after explaining the nature and cause of the problem, you might point out the strengths and weaknesses of various treatments. You might share how pets treated with a particular regimen will show improvement in about 10 days, and ask whether the client would like to try that treatment. The client is still in charge, but you have provided expert advice to help the client separate the worthwhile regimens from the worthless ones.

Use the Resources Available to You

Some clients are visual learners, others are auditory learners, and a few are tactile learners, so you should use models, dry-erase boards, radiographs, and handouts to present information in a form for all learning styles.[104,105]

About 65 percent of the population are classified as visual learners, and as the name implies, they tend to comprehend best when they are shown an image, model, or graphic that demonstrates the problem or treatment. They may need to take notes or draw their own picture to completely understand a concept.

Twenty to 25 percent of people are auditory learners—those who best assimilate the information that is shared via lecture. This statistic is important because relying on lecture alone, without using visual aids or models, may mean you're not communicating with 75 percent of your audience.

Tactile learners (10–15 percent of the population) are classic "doers." They must actually perform most tasks before they understand them, and they won't, for example, find a handout on or discussion of how to medicate the ear helpful. However, if you allow them to instill the medication in the exam room once, they'll be able to do it for the rest of their lives.[106]

Listening

Veterinarians are often so focused on delivering information that they often underuse their listening skills.[25,107] People are most satisfied with their exam room experience when they feel that the doctor was actually listening to them. Veterinarians can reassure clients that they're listening by making repeating, paraphrasing, or reflecting statements.

Repeating is essentially parroting—using exactly the same words as the client. It's the least convincing type of listening because it doesn't require much effort to repeat something. Clients may get irritated with repeating because they may misinterpret the repeated phrase as a challenge (i.e., your emphasis may imply doubt, sarcasm, or disdain, such as "You're feeding *dog chow*?")

Paraphrasing is the use of similar words or phrases in an arrangement that mirrors that of the client. In general, clients respond well to paraphrasing because it shows that you're listening to them.

Reflecting is the most complicated form of listening because it requires you to rephrase the message in your own words. The trick in the exam room is to reflect without changing the client's original message so much that he or she won't recognize it.[5,108]

Silence

In the exam room, silence is an important tool that allows the client time to form thoughts and share them with you. Asking a terrific open-ended question and then cutting the client off after one sentence doesn't accomplish anything. Your silence after asking a question shows how much you respect the client's opinion.[49]

The use of silence is also a common technique that interviewers use when they want a reluctant interviewee to tell them more.[109] People are generally uncomfortable with gaps in conversation; if the interviewer doesn't ask another question, then the interviewee will often fill the silence. Using this technique in the exam room can be illuminating, especially when you're asking a question such as "What does your dog eat?" You will likely get the standard answer, "Dog food." If you wait for about three seconds, looking at the client with an open expression on your face that says, "Tell me more," then the client will often reveal the rest of the dog's diet.[110]

Silence can also be used as a negative reinforcer if a person is speaking too much (often someone who came in with the client). If you wait silently without engaging the person (e.g., without nodding or saying "uh-huh"), he or she will eventually run out of steam.[111]

Communicating Your Findings: Problem-Oriented Exams and Risk Communication

Basically, two types of exams take place in veterinary clinics every day: wellness and problem-oriented exams. As you might expect, wellness exams involve routine vaccinations, worming, and other preventive treatments, and problem-oriented exams deal with a medical issue (or a perceived problem).

In some cases, both types of communication may occur during the same OFFICE call, such as when you've discovered a potentially serious problem during a wellness exam or if the owner is worried about a health issue that ends up being normal (e.g., bleeding gums in a puppy that is teething).

Problem-oriented exams require shifting gears and engaging in what is routinely called *risk communication*. The client's perception of risk can be one of the most challenging issues you deal with on a daily basis. In many cases, owners aren't reacting to how ill the pet really is, but to their *perception* of the severity of the problem. Acknowledging and discussing the owner's perception of a pet's problem are very important.

Peter Sandman, who has written about risk communication for more than 40 years, found that people accept risk more readily and are less fearful if the risk factors are voluntary, personally controlled, familiar, and reversible.[112] However, the level of perceived risk is high (along with fear, outrage, and dread) when the risk factors are involuntary, controlled by others, exotic, and permanent. Figure 3.3 is adapted from Peter Sandman's work.[112,113] This figure has been modified to make it more relevant to the types of risk communication seen in the veterinary setting.

Issues in the right-hand column are likely to result in stronger negative emotions (fear, outrage, dread) than those in the left-hand column. Recognizing this is important when dealing with clients who are highly emotional or angry.

Hidden Camera Simulation

Every once in a while during an exam, try to see yourself through your client's eyes, or imagine that a camera is filming you from his or her side of the room. Are you looking at the client or focusing on the chart? Are you leaning against the counter as if you're relaxed, lazy, or bored? Have you picked up the scopes (oto, ophtho, stetho) and subconsciously signaled that it is time for the visit to come to an end?

The hidden camera simulation can be enormously valuable. You may have crossed your arms simply because it was comfortable, but you are sending a clear nonverbal message that says, "I'm not receptive to you." Unfolding your arms and using a more relaxed stance will invite the client to keep talking about the pet's history.

A common scenario is the client who is convinced that a neighbor poisoned his or her dog. Although you may recognize that the dog's problem is most likely an upset stomach from too much table food, the client's level of outrage and fear makes him or her initially unreceptive to this mundane explanation. Understanding the client's emotional state allows you to speak to those issues and address the client's perception of risk. The client will be much happier if you say, "Let's run some bloodwork and see what we find," and is likely to feel dismissed (and outraged) if you say, "It's probably just a stomachache."

Enlisting with Empathy

The final stages of the OFFICE call involve enlisting clients to act and, if appropriate, showing empathy for the pet's problem and how it affects the family.

When enlisting clients to take action (e.g., approve tests, give medication), you can motivate them by appealing to their head, heart, and feet. In general, veterinarians are very good at talking to the head—for example, they will eagerly explain in a very intellectual way all of the issues associated with untreated dental disease and give a technical overview of how it can be remedied with a dental cleaning.

More empathetic colleagues recognize the importance of speaking to the heart—how a treatment plan (the dental cleaning) will affect the pet (and improve its health) and the impact on the rest of the family (e.g., the pet will be happier, more playful, and its breath will improve).

The concept of enlisting the client is critical, because this is when the owner is asked to take action.

What veterinarians don't always do well is appeal to clients' feet and ask whether they're willing to take the necessary steps to improve their pet's health—whether they involve performing bloodwork, a dental cleaning, or simply giving medication. The concept of enlisting the client is critical, because this is when the owner is asked to take action.[114,115]

FIGURE 3.3 Risk Perception and Response

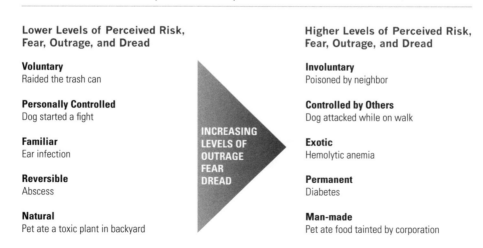

Lower Levels of Perceived Risk, Fear, Outrage, and Dread

Voluntary
Raided the trash can

Personally Controlled
Dog started a fight

Familiar
Ear infection

Reversible
Abscess

Natural
Pet ate a toxic plant in backyard

INCREASING LEVELS OF OUTRAGE FEAR DREAD

Higher Levels of Perceived Risk, Fear, Outrage, and Dread

Involuntary
Poisoned by neighbor

Controlled by Others
Dog attacked while on walk

Exotic
Hemolytic anemia

Permanent
Diabetes

Man-made
Pet ate food tainted by corporation

Adapted and modified from Sandman and Covello.[112,113]

If you've successfully appealed to the client's head, heart, and feet, then you've engaged the client on all three levels, and the chances are greater that he or she will accept and comply with the agreed-on treatment plan.

Communicating for Compliance

Acceptance (buy-in) and compliance (follow-through) both come down to the concept of perceived value—the notion that the value of a particular test, treatment, or plan is greater than its cost. The formula is simple: Perceived Value = Benefit / Cost of Delivery. Recognizing the concept of perceived value is a powerful tool in the exam room, and it will help you understand why one client says yes to a proposed plan and another says no.

The reality is that every time veterinarians recommend a vaccine, discuss a test, talk about heartworm prevention, or even offer to board a client's pets, they're engaged in some form of marketing. For clients to say yes to a diagnostic or treatment plan, they must perceive that the benefits are greater than the cost of delivery.

Benefit is determined by the client, not by the veterinarian. As the doctor, though, you may be able to help the client understand the benefit; in fact, it's an important part of your job. An X-ray of an enlarged heart and some pictures of heartworms may be enough to help an owner understand the benefit of a monthly preventive.

Cost of delivery relates to dollars and cents, but it also includes the time and trouble a particular course of action will require. For example, medicating a cat is almost never easy, so the cost is very high; therefore, the benefit needs to be even greater if the client is going to accept and comply with the treatment plan.

It's key to note that perceived value isn't a static concept that can be determined by simple math. Some clients see the need for a service or product, and others don't. The difference between these clients may be a function of their personal value system, their having tried that treatment or test before with little perceived benefit, or just not understanding why they need to buy what you're selling.[25,116]

One can apply the cost:benefit ratio to just about any situation and achieve positive results. Whether it's training a pet, motivating a staff member, or encouraging client compliance with a treatment plan, almost all people are practical enough to want to benefit from their actions—the only exception appears to be teenagers, and explaining their behavior is beyond the scope of this book.

Clients are more likely to accept and comply with a treatment plan when they personally benefit. The specific type of gain varies on the basis of the various cognitive styles, but a successful veterinarian must demonstrate benefit to all clients.[117,118]

Most veterinarians learn the hard way that clients may be angered if benefits aren't demonstrated regularly. Discussing lab work findings is an excellent example. If the client is told that the normal lab work "didn't show anything wrong," he or she is likely to think that it was a waste of money. However, if the veterinarian reports that "because the lab work was normal, we've ruled out a lot of problems—the kidneys, liver, and thyroid are working great, and your pet doesn't have any signs of anemia or an infection," the client is going to clearly see the benefit of the bloodwork.

It's essential that all members of the veterinary team learn to emphasize the benefit in a course of action when conversing with clients. When all staff members uniformly deliver the message from this perspective, clients will see the benefits in all you do!

Money Talk

The reality is that almost no office visit is complete without a discussion of the actual financial costs of the recommended tests or treatments.[119] Unfortunately, this sensitive subject is seldom touched on in an up-front manner; one study showed that fewer than one in three visits included a discussion of costs.[97]

Clients expect and need to know that you care more about their pet's health than you care about their pocketbook.[25,120] Historically, veterinarians have been guilty of demonstrating caring by devaluing and discounting their own services.[118]

It's worthwhile to remember that if you're an expert and have an expert–client relationship that is transactional, then you should expect to negotiate and barter over your fees. However, as an advisor, all you can do is present clients with the various treatment options and let them choose the plan that is acceptable to their cost:benefit ratio and pocketbook.

Empathy

Empathy is the final step in the OFFICE call, and its importance cannot be over-rated or overstated. Empathy is increasingly becoming appreciated as a critical tool in medical communication models.[87,99,121]

What is empathy? Effectively, it's understanding how a client is feeling, which differs significantly from sympathy, in which the doctor actually feels personally responsible for resolving the client's problems (see Table 3.2).[122] From a practical standpoint, doctors who display high levels of sympathy are more likely to experience burnout, depression, and decreased job satisfaction, whereas empathetic doctors have higher job satisfaction and happier clients.[123,124]

TABLE 3.2 Empathy and Sympathy

Veterinary Outlook	Empathy	Sympathy
Relationship style	Engaged detachment	Intertwined
Feelings	Feels with the client	Feels for the client
Perspective	Situation is experienced from the client's perspective	Situation is experienced from the perspective of how it would affect the doctor if roles were reversed
Responsibility	Client's responsible for choosing a solution; doctor's responsible for providing guidance and information	Doctor is fully responsible for fixing or solving the client's problems
Equality	Client is an equal	Client is deficient, needy, or deserving of pity

Adapted from Morris[122] *and Batmanabane.*[123]

In any long-term relationship, people want a partnership with someone who understands what they're feeling and why. People desire this relationship with their physicians, and loyal veterinary clients will seek the same understanding from their pet's doctor.

The misconception is that empathy is time-consuming and emotionally draining. The reality is exactly the opposite. Doctors who offer empathetic statements (e.g., "I understand how messy it is for a pet to have diarrhea for three days") save time and improve client satisfaction.[125,126] Empathy actually facilitates the process of taking a history and discussing the diagnostic or treatment plan.[127] Conversely, studies have shown that when opportunities for expressing empathy were missed, appointment times were longer and more frustrating for both the doctor and the client.[128,129]

The key steps to effective empathy are as follows:[130,131]

- Recognizing the presence of strong feelings in the exam room (anger, grief, fear, frustration)
- Stating your understanding of the client's feelings ("I imagine that must be upsetting" or "It sounds like you're worried about . . .")
- Offering support and partnership ("I'll do everything I can to help you and Sparky get through this")

Empathy is an active, verbal process. Empathy is most important when a client's level of outrage, fear, or dread (refer to earlier section, "Communicating Your Findings: Problem-Oriented Exams and Risk Communication") is at its highest, for instance when a pet has just been diagnosed with a permanent condition such as diabetes. Giving an insulin shot twice a day is not a big deal to a veterinarian, but to a client the diagnosis of a lifelong disease such as diabetes can be devastating.

By recognizing the clients' perception of the situation and restating your awareness of how they feel, empathetic doctors are respecting and legitimizing pet owners' emotions. The clients gain an understanding doctor who becomes a trusted ally. The bottom line is that empathy is good for the pets, good for the clients, and good for the veterinarian.

Two-Minute Primer on Nonverbal Communication: Posture and Body Language

Charles Darwin wrote the first book on nonverbal communication, *The Expressions of the Emotions of Man and Animals* (in 1872!).[132] Since then, nonverbal communication has been widely studied with highly variable results: Is people's body language responsible for 80 percent, 55 percent, or 93 percent of the message they deliver, or only 20 percent?[‡,75,76,81,83,85,133,134] It doesn't really matter what the percentage is; what matters is that veterinarians recognize and accept that nonverbal communication is a significant component of what they say even when they're not saying anything.

Although much of nonverbal communication seems obvious and intuitive, it is amazing how many unintended messages people send with their body language. Here's a quick overview of those that are most useful in the exam room.

Attentive Body Language

Through body posture and position, veterinarians can send a clear message to clients that they are interested in the pet and what clients have to say.[135] Many veterinarians don't realize when they've adopted inattentive body language, but clients certainly recognize it.[136]

- **Ignoring distractions:** For the client to feel valued, it is important for the veterinarian to remain focused on the client and the pet in the exam room. Reacting to stimuli outside the exam room suggests that the veterinarian is not completely engaged (e.g., responding to a ringing cell phone or something that is overheard outside of the exam room). This also means that distractions—such as constant interruptions by the staff during an OFFICE call—aren't allowed.

- **Remaining still:** Nervous fidgeting and looking around are clear signs of impatience or inattention.

- **Leaning forward:** Leaning forward indicates an interest in what the client is saying.

- **Turning the top of the body:** Turning your body toward the person to whom you want to speak can be helpful, especially when the client has brought in a friend who won't be quiet. By turning toward the client and away from the talkative friend, you signal that it is the client's opportunity to talk.

- **Tilting head:** Tilting your head forward suggests interest. Tilting your head sideways may indicate curiosity or confusion. Tilting the head down to look at the client may be viewed as condescending or judgmental. Note that people who tilt their head down to look over the top of their bifocals may be sending an unintentionally negative message.

- **Gaze:** When you look directly at the speaker, you're showing an interest in what he or she has to say. This is important for those veterinarians who write all of their medical notes while the client is talking.

continues

Two-Minute Primer on Nonverbal Communication: Posture and Body Language, continued

- **Furrowed brow:** A furrowed brow implies you are concentrating on what the person is saying.

- **Open body:** Holding your arms open and at your sides, putting your hands in your pockets, and not crossing your legs tightly (if you are sitting) are open and encouraging. Many veterinarians stand with their arms crossed for comfort, which actually sends a negative nonverbal message.

- **Slow nodding:** Slow nodding encourages the speaker to tell you more.

- **Encouraging words:** Saying "uh-huh" and "hmmm" also shows that you are engaged.137

- **Reflecting body language:** When your pose is similar to that of the speaker, you're matching his or her mood on a subconscious level.

Bored or Disinterested Body Language

Although no veterinarian would purposely send bored or disinterested signals to a paying client, it's worth doing a self-assessment from time to time and making sure that you aren't guilty of one of these infractions.

- **Distraction:** Looking around the room, checking the time on the clock, doodling.

- **Repeated movements:** Toe-tapping, drumming fingers, clicking a pen.

- **Fatigue:** Yawning, slouching, sagging against the wall, an inexpressive face, which will shut down almost any client.

- **Et cetera:** Essentially, the opposite of the nonverbal cues in the "Attentive Body Language" section.

Dominant Body Language

If clients are already nervous in the veterinary setting, any type of dominant body language will further intimidate them.[136] Awareness of one's body posture and position in relation to the client will help prevent any unintended dominant messages from being sent.

- **Making the body big:** Hands on hips, chest out, chin up, and legs apart. You may put your hands on your hips because it's a comfortable resting place, but do clients feel pressured if you do this while making a recommendation regarding their pet?

- **Standing tall:** Taking the high ground and looking down on your client. Standing tall is clearly a dominant posture. Tall veterinarians should always have a stool or chair in the exam room where they can sit at eye level with the client and talk.

- **Occupying territory:** Moving into the client's personal space, for example.

- **Breaking rules of etiquette:** Interrupting the speaker using inappropriate and potentially offensive language.

Conclusion

Effective exam room communication goes beyond simply explaining the nature of a pet's problem to clients. Speaking with warm vocal tones, making small talk, and using respectful silences can enhance the client's exam room experience. Nonverbal communication also plays an important role, because the veterinarian's body language also sends important messages to the pet owner.

The OFFICE call system emphasizes the importance of first impressions, friendly talk, enlisting the client to act, and empathy. Smiling and displaying a non-anxious presence are key from the outset of the OFFICE call and will make clients feel valued and appreciated.

OFFICE calls can be divided into wellness exams and problem-oriented exams. Problem-oriented exams require a shift of communication gears—and veterinarians must understand the fundamental aspects of risk communication when discussing problems with pet owners.

Notes

*"Based on hundreds of interviews I've conducted on this subject with both senior corporate executives and individual advisors, it's clear that there are three main drivers of client loyalty: 1) The value you add, 2) The degree of trust you develop, and 3) Going the extra mile."[102]

†Author unknown.

‡A frequent misinterpretation of the study referenced in Milani that has become "nonverbal gospel."[46]

§Reflective listening, empathy, nonverbal communication, open-ended questions.

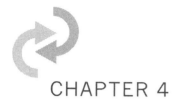

CHAPTER 4

Grief Communication and Euthanasia

When it comes to end-of-life discussions, veterinarians wear multiple hats: unbiased doctor, advocate for the animal, and therapist to the client. The greater the family's attachment to an animal, the greater the veterinarian's stress regarding discussion of and decisions about euthanasia. This is no small problem: The moral stress associated with euthanasia is the most significant cause of job dissatisfaction among veterinarians.[138]

For clients, attachment to a pet seems to vary depending on their life stage (see Figure 4.1). The lowest levels of attachment are seen in households with infant children; middle amounts of attachment, in homes with elementary-school-age or teenage children; and higher levels of attachment, in empty nesters, newlyweds, and remarried couples. The highest level of attachment is seen in divorced, never married, or childless couples and elderly widowed people.[139]

Emotion at losing a pet is a normal human reaction and is seen at all levels of pet ownership. Men rated a pet's death as similar to the loss of a close friend, and

FIGURE 4.1 Levels of Attachment to Pets

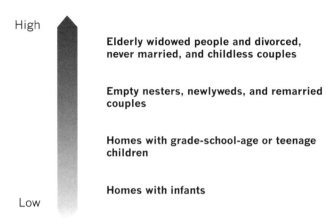

women tended to rate the emotional loss as being on par with losing touch with a child. One-half of all women surveyed and more than one-quarter of all men said that the loss of their pet was quite or extremely disturbing.[140]

Veterinarians know that euthanasia is emotionally difficult, but who knew it was that stressful?

The Euthanasia Visit

In the clinic setting, there are predominantly three types of euthanasia visits: *expected, impulsive,* and *unexpected.* Each situation provides its own unique type of stress, but they share some common challenges:[141,142]

- Seeing euthanasia as a failure
- Worrying that others will make a value judgment about the care the owners provided for their pet (i.e., that they didn't do enough or are making the wrong decision)
- Inherent discomfort with death's finality
- Losing the pet's companionship

- Beginning of a grieving process[143,144]

From the doctor's perspective, the challenges of euthanasia include the following:

- Determining whether euthanasia is the humane choice
- Helping clients manage their grief (grief is a normal reaction to any sort of loss,[145] and the death of a pet is almost always very difficult for most people)
- Maintaining a positive relationship with the client for other or future animals
- Euthanizing the animal with a minimum of added stress and a maximum of kindness
- Being concerned about euthanasia being seen as a treatment failure
- Being concerned about highly emotional clients or those in the anger phase taking out their frustration by threatening litigation or license review
- Working through the euthanasia appointment quickly enough to stay on schedule and getting paid for the service

How do you overcome these barriers to good communication? Relying on the basics of exam room communication will help, specifically the information on being an advisor, listening, discussing crisis and risk management, and using empathy. You also must create a supportive environment for the euthanasia discussion. For these talks, you should have a comfortable, quiet room, free of interruptions from your staff. There isn't a right or a particular way in which to experience grief, so be ready for a number of different reactions by pet owners. Being aware of the stages of grief (see the sidebar "The Five Stages of Grief") can help you prepare for these conversations. Finally, knowing whether it is an expected, impulsive, or unexpected euthanasia will help you figure out the best way to conduct the initial conversation and what emotional responses to expect.

Expected Euthanasia

In an expected euthanasia, the owner has had some time to prepare for the animal's death, so denial is not an issue. Two key elements to creating a positive bond

The Five Stages of Grief

According to Elisabeth Kübler-Ross, there are five stages of grief.[144,145]

- **Denial:** My cat can't have kidney failure; she was just eating the other day.
- **Anger:** If you were a good doctor, you would find the cause.
- **Bargaining:** Can't we just give her some sort of supplement? I found one on the Internet.
- **Depression:** I'm really going to miss her. I'm never going to get another cat.
- **Acceptance:** What do I need to do to keep her happy as long as possible?

Note: Not all people feel all stages, and the stages do not occur in any particular order.

between you and a client when performing a euthanasia are (1) acknowledging that the owner is making the right decision and (2) expressing sorrow and empathy for the client's loss. If you don't express these emotions in some way when you perform a euthanasia, you could risk angering the client and may increase your risk of litigation. Some clients are still in the anger stage when they arrive for the anticipated euthanasia, and it's important to work through the process with them and move them closer to the acceptance stage.

Impulsive Euthanasia

The impulsive euthanasia is generally seen with a walk-in appointment or an owner who insists on getting into the clinic that day. These owners are often reacting to a negative behavior that the pet keeps exhibiting; two of the most common scenarios are a dog that is biting and a cat that is soiling the house.

The key to resolving an impulsive euthanasia is to determine what problem the pet poses for the owner and then to see whether the owner is interested in pursuing a remedy to that problem. You can then negotiate with the owner about the possible choices for rehabilitation or correction.

For example, perhaps a pet's bad behavior has caused the owner to snap, and he or she doesn't want to put up with it anymore. This situation requires a lot of finesse, because the owner is dealing with several strong emotions: anger or frustration with the situation and resentment at having to make this decision. Some family members may not support the decision, and the owner may be expecting a backlash along with an unpleasant grieving process once he or she gets home.

It's important to talk with the owner and ask why he or she wants the pet euthanized.[146] This talk should, of course, occur in the privacy of the exam room, because the owner may already feel judged by family members and won't want to be judged by strangers as well.

You may think that the pet has a chance to be rehabilitated, and this is where it gets tricky. Instead of making value judgments, it's best to solicit the client's impression of the situation. For example, you could ask, "Do you think that with training he might stop biting?" or "Is it possible that extra litter boxes and some anxiety medication might help with the house soiling?"

If the client opens the door and wants to know more about behavior modification, then you have an invitation to try and rehabilitate the pet. If the owner doesn't want to rehabilitate the animal, but you think it's a diamond in the rough, then you may approach the subject of a rescue group or the Society for Prevention of Cruelty to Animals.

In some cases, the pet may have a physical problem (e.g., a large tumor), and the owner has assumed that it can't be fixed or will be too costly to repair. Refer to the section "Enlisting and Empathy" in Chapter 3, and its subsection, "Money Talk," for some tips on discussing the value of surgery with this client.

If the client refuses these options and doesn't want more information, then you'll need to make a decision as to whether you are morally opposed to euthanizing the pet.[147] Before stating this moral opposition, you should first reflect on the realities of the situation and consider both the animal and the owner:[148–150]

- The client may have many more reasons for requesting the pet's euthanasia than originally stated (e.g., the client can't afford to feed his or her family, let alone the pet; the client is losing his or her house and the backyard where the animal lived; the pet has additional behavior or health problems).

- Owners have the legal right to choose the relationship they have with their animals.
- It may be extremely stressful for the pet to be placed in a new home.
- Someone else may not provide this animal with as humane a death as you can.
- For many reasons, veterinarians simply cannot save all of the pets they encounter.

If, after this reflection, you still cannot euthanize the animal, then you need to consult with other doctors in the practice and determine whether they feel differently. If they are similarly opposed to euthanizing the animal, then you must apologize to the client, explain that you simply cannot perform the procedure because you feel it would violate your oath to help animals, and offer the client referrals to rescue groups or specialists. It is best to be clear, direct, and compassionate with language. Here is some sample language:

> *I know that this is a difficult situation, but I have to be honest with you about this. Ethically, I cannot and will not perform the euthanasia you've requested. I can work with you on exploring other options if you'd like, but if not, you'll need to consult with another veterinarian. I'm sorry that I can't help you.*

It is best to immediately refund any fees that the client has paid while he or she is still in the exam room. Although this situation will no doubt have been time-consuming for you, moral dilemmas are emotionally charged, and this is not a time to quibble about money.

Unexpected Euthanasia (or Death)

The unexpected euthanasia or death is the most challenging end-of-life situation of all, because the owner has not had any time to process the severity of the problem. These cases are often seen either in emergency situations or in hospitalized patients that took an unforeseen turn for the worse.

The unexpected euthanasia creates an emotionally difficult atmosphere in which denial and anger are likely seen. Certainly, all veterinarians try to minimize the unexpected in the course of their day, but treating sick animals isn't the same as tuning an engine—and not all pets get better in spite of your best efforts.

If possible, it's best to meet with the owners before euthanizing the pet. They need to be aware of the pet's issues. After the discussion, give them a chance to visit with the pet for a while and come back to answer any questions they have. Take your time with these clients; they need to see your thoughtfulness and caring. The few times that I've felt physically threatened in the clinic have stemmed from anger over unexpected deaths. Taking your time can defuse the situation.

Not every unexpected death has to be unexpected. Fortunately, it doesn't take a lot of forewarning to move from unexpected to expected. Calling an owner while CPR is being performed on their pet will allow them to begin processing the possibility that their pet may die. In fact, even if you call the owner 15 minutes later with bad news, the backlash isn't nearly as great.

If the pet unexpectedly died in the clinic, then offer to meet with the owner later that day (when you won't be hurried) to have a discussion about the euthanasia or death. The owner needs to know the sequence of events, what happened, how you reacted, and why it didn't work.

Naturally, clients aren't happy when their pet dies unexpectedly or suddenly becomes so ill that it must be euthanized, but your concern and your taking the time to explain the situation to them will maintain their trust in you. For more in-depth information on communicating with clients in moments of grief or other conflicts, refer to the AAHA Press publication *Connecting with Clients: Practical Communication for 10 Common Situations*, Second Edition.[151,*]

Conclusion

End-of-life discussions are among the most challenging aspects of veterinary practice. Coping with the various emotions of pet owners as they process grief (e.g., anger, denial, depression) can be difficult and time-consuming, yet it is important for the veterinarian to accept this challenge.

Handled well, an end-of-life discussion can bond a client to your practice; but poorly managed, it will almost certainly create client dissatisfaction or anger, and may even trigger litigation. With good communication, however, you ensure that you are counseling a pet owner about euthanasia in a supportive, empathetic environment conducive to appropriate decisions being made for the pet.

Note

*For more helpful information on resolving exam-room conflicts specific to veterinarians, refer to the following articles: "Difficult interactions with veterinary clients: Working in the challenge zone" by James K. Morrisey, DVM, and Bonia Voiland, MS, MBA; and "Disclosing medical errors: Restoring client trust" by Kathleen A. Bonvicini, EdD, MPH, Daniel O'Connell, PhD, and Karen K. Cornell, DVM, PhD, DACVS.

PART TWO

The Art of Conversing with Clients

Clients have difficulty determining whether a doctor is competent, but they are experts on whether that doctor has communicated with them effectively.[152] In this section, we emphasize the importance of "conversation" as a form of communication. By definition, conversation is a two-way and interactive process.[153] The key to improving a conversation is "talking each other's language," which has been shown to dramatically improve medical outcomes.[154] Conversation style is a function of an individual's personality, so understanding how a person thinks and interacts with the world is key to speaking their language.[155–158]

Of course, people come in a variety of shapes, sizes, and personalities. Just like the leopard's spots, no two people are exactly the same. Yet, people's personality styles can be identified, labeled, and assigned to various categories.

Some of the earliest known work on personality styles was done before Plato and Hippocrates, by Ezekiel in 590 BC, and the study of human behavior has continued throughout written history. Interestingly, most of these approaches, although derived independently, classify people into four different personality styles (also called sources of happiness, worldviews, and goals).[159]

In this part of the book, I modify and redefine some of the modern concepts of personality classification, based on these assessments:

- Myers-Briggs Type Indicator[160–163]
- Keirsey Temperament Sorter[164,165]
- Communication Assessment Tool[42]
- Lens of Understanding[166]
- Reid and Merrill's social styles[49,167]

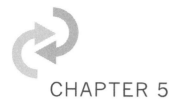

CHAPTER 5

Cognitive and Social Styles

Building on the substantial communication literature cited in the introduction of Part Two, this section of the book identifies four distinct social styles (Leader, Engineer, Energizer, Dreamer) and four specific cognitive styles (Hawk, Dog, Kitten, Owl). In brief, social style describes how you interact with others, and cognitive style identifies how you perceive and process information.[160–163] The four social and four cognitive styles result in 16 possible personality type combinations (e.g., Leader Hawk or Dreamer Dog).

Although most people have one preferred social style and one preferred cognitive style, their personality is a composite of these 16 preferences (see Table 5.1).[42,160,161,163] In other words, people's personality is like a house with 16 rooms, with one room being the most comfortable and the best furnished. Although people aren't locked into only one room, substantial research has shown that most people do prefer one social-cognitive style combination.[168] However, people can and will visit the other rooms from time to time.

Some people actually adopt a specific social-cognitive style at home and a different one at work! For example, the naturally quiet and reserved veterinarian must visit the social parts of his or her personality house every day in the clinic—because a successful veterinary practitioner must communicate with the pet owner.

TABLE 5.1 Social-Cognitive Style Combinations

Cognitive Style	Social Style			
	Leader	Engineer	Energizer	Dreamer
Hawk	Leader Hawk	Engineer Hawk	Energizer Hawk	Dreamer Hawk
Dog	Leader Dog	Engineer Dog	Energizer Dog	Dreamer Dog
Kitten	Leader Kitten	Engineer Kitten	Energizer Kitten	Dreamer Kitten
Owl	Leader Owl	Engineer Owl	Energizer Owl	Dreamer Owl

Here's another way to look at preferred social and cognitive styles: Write your name on a piece of paper. Now put the pen in your other hand and write your name. I'm sure you can do it, but is it how you prefer to write your name? Over time and with practice, you undoubtedly could adapt to writing with your opposite hand, and that adaptability is the essence of personality types: You may prefer a certain social-cognitive style combination, but you can still develop many of the other aspects of your personality.

Social Style: How People Interact

Social style isn't simply a measure of whether you are talkative or a wallflower. Instead, social style is a combination of your sociability (outgoing or reserved) and your willingness to make decisions (decisive or open-ended; see Table 5.2). As you know, people's personalities are incredibly complex. This book distills the major studies on personality, including *Gifts Differing, Type Talk at Work, The Art of Speed Reading People, Please Understand Me II,* and *Leveraging Your*

Communication Style, to identify the four social styles as Leaders, Engineers, Energizers, and Dreamers.[42,160,161,164] Besides simplifying the social styles and terminology in the cited references, this book also interprets the personality combinations in a unique manner within the context of the veterinary world.

TABLE 5.2 Four Attitudes

Decisiveness	Sociability	
	Outgoing	Reserved
Decisive	Leader	Engineer
Open-ended	Energizer	Dreamer

Leaders

These folks are outgoing and decisive. They are influential and often find themselves overseeing or coaching others to success. Of course, Leaders are going to take charge, so someone had better follow! Keirsey noted that people in this category are "directive and expressive" and referred to them as *teachers, field marshals,* and *supervisors.*[165,169] Allen and Brock wrote that Leaders are "decisive, [and] quickly move to implement decisions."[163]

Engineers

Reserved but decisive, Engineers quietly observe their world and make few suggestions—but you should listen when they speak, because they have great insight. Engineers tend to focus on specific details or situations, so they aren't trying to change the entire world—just their part of it. According to Keirsey, Engineers may be thought of as counselors, masterminds, and inspectors.[165] *Type Talk at Work* says that Engineers are "life's natural organizers" and display "scholarly dependability."[161]

Energizers

These outgoing people are always engaging others and tinkering with the status quo (or, some might say, "stirring the pot"), trying to make things better, get things done, and create variety. When it comes to decision making, Energizers are open-ended, so the rules can (and often do) change on a regular basis. Aptly named, Energizers are action-oriented and tend to spur others to action as well. Synonyms for Energizers include *promoters, performers*, and *champions*.[165] Berens et al. referred to Energizers as "motivators, explorers, and discoverers."[162]

Dreamers

Reserved and open-ended, Dreamers may seem aloof, but they're actually thinking about ways to improve everyone's quality of life. Dreamers aren't going to rock the boat most days, unless their personal value system is threatened—and then watch out! Dreamers may also be called *healers, architects, crafters,* and *composers*.[165]

Cognitive Style: How People Perceive and Process

The concept of cognitive style is often misunderstood. In psychological terms, cognition isn't a determination of brainpower or intelligence; instead, it refers to innate aspects (or preferences) of personality—specifically, how people gather information about the world and how they use that information to make decisions.[57,170] In subsequent chapters, I explore these four cognitive styles at length and provide you with the means to identify which type of client you are talking to in the exam room. (See Table 5.3.)

In the veterinary exam room, cognitive style is "where the rubber meets the road." Understanding clients' cognitive style (how they understand and act on what the doctor is saying) is essential to successfully conversing with them, whereas knowing whether they are comfortable speaking in front of the local Rotary Club (i.e., social style) is not.[163,166]

TABLE 5.3 Four Temperaments

Decision Making	Information Gathering	
	Data and Facts	Abstract and Intuitive
Logical and mathematical	Hawk	Owl
Emotional and empathetic	Dog	Kitten

How clients process information and make decisions ultimately affects how they prefer to communicate. Identifying clients' cognitive style doesn't diminish their individuality in any way; instead, it gives you a powerful framework with which to begin to understand the people you encounter on a daily basis.

> *Identifying clients' cognitive style doesn't diminish their individuality . . . instead, it gives you a powerful framework with which to begin to understand the people you encounter on a daily basis.*

Again, this book modifies, simplifies, and redefines some of the modern concepts of personality types and the understanding of cognitive styles, and is based on several popular references in this area, including *Gifts Differing, Talk Type at Work, Please Understand Me II, Lens of Understanding,* and *Leveraging Your Communication Style.*[42,160,161,165,166]

Hawks

Hawks combine fact-based information gathering and logical decision making. Hawks get their information by interacting with the physical world—using their senses to see and hear all that is around them. With that information, they then make a decision in a logical and impersonal manner. Hawks ask, "What's the bottom line?" and "What's in it for me?" They aren't uncaring robots; they just don't need or want all of that touchy-feely stuff to make their best decisions. A Hawk is efficient and goal-oriented.

Dogs

Dogs combine fact-based information gathering and empathetic decision making. They get their information through their senses (they need real-world data, not just theories or ideas) and will consider who is affected by their decisions. Dogs are most interested in relationships—with their pets and with you. Dogs are practical. Although they want personalized recommendations, they are also the first to ask, "How have others dealt with this?" They don't like logic without feeling.

Kittens

Kittens combine abstract information gathering and empathetic decision making. Kittens think that life should just be experienced. They make decisions by considering the feelings of all involved. Kittens are "live-and-let-live" types and care more about the journey than the destination. These pet owners are all about the fun that their pet brings, and they want to understand the big picture, not the nuts and bolts. They don't react well to pressure or lectures and instead want to emphasize harmony and quality of life.

Owls

Owls combine abstract information gathering and logical decision making. Owls live in a world of ideas and logic. They seek patterns and understanding. They are ingenious and problem solving by nature. Owls don't take things at face value and are skeptical. It isn't that they doubt you—they simply doubt everything they're told and constantly challenge the conventions of what is known. They like looking at the long term and will ask questions about things that seem far off in the distance.

Conclusion

Throughout written history, scholars have been trying to group others in terms of cognitive and social styles. Although all people are complicated creatures, they tend to adopt one of four social styles (Leader, Engineer, Energizer, Dreamer) and one of four cognitive styles (Hawk, Dog, Owl, Kitten). Social style is determined by an individual's sociability and decisiveness, whereas cognitive style is a function of a person's preferred information sources and decision-making processes.

CHAPTER 6

Determining Cognitive Style

Cognitive style refers to how an individual gathers information and makes decisions with it. Understanding clients' cognitive style in the exam room is more important than understanding their social style because you're presenting them with information and asking them to make decisions. When veterinarians speak to clients in their cognitive style, the likelihood that communication and outcomes will be enhanced is greater because they are "speaking the clients' language."

How People Gather Information

In general, people fall into one of two groups: Either they need specific and detailed information to make decisions, or they are more intuitive and don't require facts and data.[42,160,163]

Data-Driven and Fact-Based Information Gathering

Some people must see, taste, hear, touch, or smell something to know that it exists. In other words, they need data and facts. In the exam room, Hawks and Dogs, who are data-driven and fact-based, tend to do the following:

- Ask practical questions
- Want a step-by-step approach or analysis
- Be excellent observers of their pet's condition and problems
- Want to know what or who else
- Focus on the details
- Prefer to live in the present
- Want to take the tried-and-true approach to diagnosing or treating their pet's problem

Abstract and Intuitive Information Gathering

Kittens and Owls, who are abstract and intuitive clients, ponder the alternatives and are fueled by intuition. They'll make mental leaps during your explanation of their pet's problem—sometimes coming out of nowhere with a question that might be brilliant or absurd. Kittens and Owls tend to do the following:

- Ask "why" questions
- Know that something is wrong with their pet without having specifics
- Want to look at the big picture
- Look at the data and try to come up with alternative explanations
- Want to blaze their own trail in pursuing a treatment or diagnostic plan

How People Make Decisions

How do clients use information to make a decision? Do they follow a tried-and-true logical or mathematical approach, or do they think more empathetically and ask how this decision will affect others?

Almost everyone combines logic and empathy when making decisions—so logical deciders aren't coldhearted machines and empathetic deciders aren't weak-kneed pushovers. Yet, people do tend to prefer one approach over the other (logic or empathy) when making a decision.[42,160,163]

Logical Decision Makers

Some people are primarily governed by logic, which means they are more comfortable making decisions that don't involve feelings. A logical thinker will do an excellent job of designing a floor plan for your veterinary clinic but will be challenged when making a tough, emotional decision about whether to put an ailing pet through chemotherapy. Logical clients will deal with their pet's cancer by discussing the survival rates, the side effects of chemotherapy treatments, and the cost. With that information, they will decide if it's worth it.

Logical-thinking clients (Hawks and Owls) tend to do the following:

- Be more straightforward and less tactful
- Seem curt, businesslike, and less friendly
- Ignore or dismiss discussions about feelings that they can't process in a logical way
- Habitually question the standard conclusions that are made

This preference does have a gender bias, with two-thirds of men being Hawks or Owls.[160] Again, this doesn't mean that Hawks or Owls are heartless robots—they're just less comfortable dealing with the emotional aspects of a situation and more comfortable thinking about the pluses and minuses of a problem.

Empathetic Decision Makers

Although people in this group can and do make logical decisions, their process is less grounded in logic and more in tune with the sentimental or emotional implications of the decision. Empathetic clients (Dogs and Kittens) tend to do the following:

- Be more social and friendly
- Not present information in a linear way and seem to ramble at times
- Accept the information they are given
- Want to spend more time talking about general topics and be less focused on the task at hand

- Take feelings into account when making a decision and need more than just the cold, hard facts

Dogs or Kittens will show a greater interest in the individuals involved with a situation than in the specifics. In the case of the pet that needs chemotherapy, a Dog or Kitten will weigh the benefits against how the pet will feel while receiving treatment, the value of extending the pet's life, and the importance of the pet to the family. Across the United States, about two-thirds of all Dogs or Kittens are women.[160]

Logic, Empathy, and Intelligence

It's important to note that logical deciders aren't more intelligent than empathetic deciders. In fact, intelligence tests seem to place a higher premium on abstract information gathering (Kitten and Owl tendencies) than on logical information gathering—and many Kittens, with the cognitive style that combines abstract information gathering and empathetic decision making, have the highest IQ scores.[171]

Conclusion

As you have seen, people have a preferred way of gathering information (data-driven or intuitive) and a preferred way of making decisions (logical or empathetic). When gathering information, Hawks and Dogs are data-driven and fact-based. Owls and Kittens are intuitive. In terms of decision making, Hawks and Owls are logical, whereas Kittens and Dogs are more empathetic.

CHAPTER 7

The Hawk

Imagine a hawk soaring high in the air. A model of efficiency, the hawk flaps its wings only when necessary, letting the air currents carry it along. The hawk acts when it sees the need—something tasty is scurrying around on the ground, and the hawk moves with full speed to acquire it.

Hawks at a Glance

Driving Force: Accuracy, Efficiency, Accountability, and Benefit

Hawks are very literal people. They don't live in an abstract world; what they see is what they get. Hawks approach pet care almost mathematically—it's not that they don't care about their pet, but your proposals will need to make sense *and* cents.

Motto: "The Shortest Distance Between Two Points Is a Straight Line"

Hawks want the facts and nothing but the facts. Hawks respond well to discussions about your experience or the latest study. They don't like experiments. In complicated cases, it's important that you map out for them the route you are going to take to a diagnosis. Hawks want if-then statements: If the test shows this, then we'll treat it this way.

Conversation Style: Straightforward, Based on Observable Fact

In the more extreme cases, Hawks' conversation style may seem impersonal. In most instances, however, they recognize that they'll have a limited amount of time to spend in an exam room, and they want to maximize the information shared.

Need Information to Be: Brief, Sequential, Relevant, and Honest

Hawks are all about data and logic. They want the information presented in a coherent fashion. Your clarity equals your competence. Hawks appreciate it when you use the dry-erase board to give your discussion an outline or a foundation.

Want to Know: What and How? What Will Be Gained? What Will It Cost? How Will the Results Be Used?

Hawks don't need to understand the finer points of how you draw blood, but they want to know what you'll do with the results—if you're drawing blood without a reason, then that's a waste of time and money. Explain how a test adds to the general understanding of a pet's condition by ruling in or ruling out certain types of diseases.

Become Angry When: Costs Exceed Estimates, Unforeseen Complications or Reactions Occur, Agreements Aren't Honored

Hawks don't like surprises. A pet that takes an unexpected turn for the worse while under your care is going to be a problem. If you think a Hawk's pet isn't responding as it should, you need to communicate this. Any advance warning and preparation will allow Hawks to process the new data and update their view of the situation.

With Hawks, your word is your bond. If you say you'll call on Monday with laboratory results, then you'd better call on Monday.

Serious Medical Problems

Hawks don't do the unknown very well. It's more important to emphasize what you do know and what you've been able to rule out and to provide a flowchart for the next tests that need to be run. Provide a step-by-step plan, and they'll be more comfortable. Hawks live in a logical, cause-and-effect world. When problems occur (such as a pet that seems critically ill overnight), they may become mired in the cause. Help them focus on the effect, because that's what you're treating, but it's important for them to see that you are pursuing the cause as well (which you would do anyway).

Emergencies

With the most inflexible cognitive style, Hawks hate emergencies. They may act outraged (outgoing Leaders and Energizers) or catatonic (reserved Engineers and Dreamers). Give them time to process the information, and provide them with a game plan. Be honest, and deal with Hawks as straightforwardly as possible by providing them with facts. In an emotionally charged situation such as an emergency, any additional drama will make things worse.

Money

Hawks are generally very aware of their financial situation and may be very up-front about what they can and can't afford. In some cases, this admission of financial constraints may be the opening round of a negotiation. It's up to you to determine what's best for the pet and present it to the owner. Hawks typically prefer a couple of treatment plan options, and they don't always opt for the least expensive of the two. When Hawks opt for a less involved plan, you need to put the responsibility of observation and communication on them—it's up to them to bring the pet back if it doesn't respond to the treatment plan. This strategy works well with Hawks because they are into observing their world.

Euthanasia and Grief

Hawks may seem a little cold or clinical about decisions such as euthanasia, but that doesn't mean they make those decisions lightly. There's little doubt that they've weighed the available information and come up with the conclusion that euthanasia is best. If you've never seen this client before, then there might be an opportunity to help the pet; for example, perhaps the pet is a dog with arthritis that will respond to anti-inflammatory medications. You can tell the Hawk, "I can see why you've made this tough decision today. [pause] Sometimes there are treatments for this that might help, but I'd need to do some tests." Some Hawk clients will want to hear more, and others won't.

The Difficult Client

If a Hawk is being particularly difficult, he or she may be having issues in some other part of his or her life. An underlying financial problem or interpersonal conflict may be clouding the Hawk's normally analytical judgment (e.g., it's the spouse's dog, and they're divorcing). In some cases, the problem is that the Hawk doesn't understand what is wrong with the pet, which causes the uncertainty that a Hawk finds so troubling. Remember, Hawks are data-driven and fact-based—not having information is extremely troubling to people with this cognitive style. Provide the Hawk with data and details, and you'll have a client who is much more pleasant to work with.

If you're being tested by a Hawk, it may mean the following:

- You look too young to know what you're talking about. If you're a new graduate and are frustrated by this, don't worry—you'll look older soon enough. Try to take it with a sense of humor and professionalism.
- You have not established your credibility. Perhaps you're new to the practice, or you came in seeming distracted, or maybe you asked the same question twice and the client is wondering if you're even listening. Start from scratch if you need to, and rephrase the information you've been given so that the client knows you're engaged with him or her and the pet's problems.

- Your presentation is too scattered for the client to understand. He or she wants statistics, percentages, experience, and a structured framework.

Special Considerations with Social-Cognitive Style Combinations
Leader Hawks

The outgoing, talkative Leader Hawk tends to be a difficult client. These folks are used to being in charge, and it's difficult for them to give up control and let you run the show. You can help the situation by consulting them each time a test is performed and talking about what the next steps are going to be.

Leader Hawks also tend to be very decisive and organized. Once a decision is made, they expect everyone to fall into line. This client will be outwardly angry if you don't perform as expected (e.g., call when you say you're going to, run the test that was agreed on). Of course, apologize if you didn't hold up your end of the bargain—and then do better next time. If the pet takes an unforeseen turn for the worse, the Leader Hawk is likely to be shocked or outraged. It's up to you to provide a context for the sudden change in the pet's condition, so the Leader Hawk can fit it back into his or her organized world.

Energizer Hawks

These owners bring a lot of energy into the exam room. They'll drop a week's worth of information on you in about five minutes, and it's up to you to assimilate it all.

Energizer Hawks want to do something proactive to solve the pet's problem. They won't be comfortable with a let's-wait-and-see approach, but they'll require that you pursue only treatments that have a high benefit:cost ratio.

Energizers tend to be more open-ended when making decisions, so they handle sudden changes with more tolerance than their Leader counterparts, but they still don't like surprises. This open-ended nature can make them less decisive, however, so Energizer Hawks like to go over the data several times (perhaps endlessly) before they decide on a course of action for you to take.

Engineer and Dreamer Hawks

These clients tend to be quieter, contemplative, or more withdrawn. You'll need to create a sense that there's plenty of time to address their pet's issues. If they think you're hassled or harried, they'll shut down. The bottom line is, if you don't have the time to hear all of the data they need to share, then they don't see the point in sharing any of it.

Engineer and Dreamer Hawks love written information—they'll assimilate everything you put in front of them.[172] They'll actually read it and appreciate it when you point out that your phone number is on the page if they have any questions.

Engineer Hawks

Engineer Hawks are very traditional in their approach to everything; they'll opt for the typical diagnostic or treatment plan. They're not going to take the road less traveled.

Engineer Hawks do love data—and they may present you with either a detailed journal of their observations of the pet or several pages of information that they downloaded from the Internet. Even if it doesn't seem pertinent, you should look at the information they've assembled. If you take Engineers' information seriously, then you're taking them seriously.

If you take Engineers' information seriously, then you're taking them seriously.

Like all Hawks, Engineer Hawks will be particularly troubled if their pet takes a sudden turn for the worse, although they'll be less likely to be confrontational than their more outgoing counterparts.

Dreamer Hawks

Dreamer Hawks tend to watch the pet a bit longer to make certain that it's really sick. They're likely to test the pet's upset stomach (in a case of gastroenteritis) and offer a buffet of tasty treats. If the pet doesn't pass the test, then they're on their way to the clinic. Of all the Hawks, Dreamer Hawks are the most theoretical because they're open-ended in how they make life's decisions.

Dreamer Hawks are one of the least engaging personality types; they're so reserved and detail-oriented that they don't really seem to want to interact with the veterinarian. This can make them appear Owlish at times. Don't confuse their lukewarm responses with dislike or disinterest; Dreamer Hawks are simply more comfortable "conversing" with a database than with a real person.

Some Hawks You May Meet

Spartan

As you may remember from history class, the Spartans were members of a Greek city-state that sacrificed most luxuries to support its military. Sparta was the dominant military force in ancient Greece for much of its existence. A Spartan's lifestyle was free from superficial and unnecessary comforts.

The client who is a Spartan will be simply and functionally dressed and will have a no-frills dog—probably a working dog of some sort. If the dog's collar is any fancier than twine, someone else bought it.

This client is most likely at your clinic because of a pressing need—for example, a laceration, bleeding tumor, or eye injury. Don't take it personally; Spartans are penny-pinchers in every aspect of their lives and believe that everyone is trying to sell them something they don't need. Spartans' goal is to attend to their pet's immediate needs. They're not interested in fancy tests or good-smelling shampoos, just the basics. Don't try selling them anything—they're not buying. Instead, discuss the low price of treatment versus the high cost later of not treating, and let them do the math.

When making recommendations, it's best to first go through the physical exam and narrate your findings as you proceed. Don't make recommendations at this point—just mention the gingivitis and gum recession, for example, and move on with the exam. Take time to discuss the good things that you see about the pet (nice coat, well behaved, etc.). Spartans will be thinking, "Hey, the doctor's spent 10 minutes looking at my pet, and hasn't even tried to sell me anything—maybe she's all right!" At this point, Spartans will be a little more receptive to talking about the problems you've noted during the pet's physical exam. This is a good time to mention the value of vaccinations or discuss flea control, dental disease, and so on.

Apathetic

Apathetic clients just don't care. They're disengaged from your universe. Apathetic clients usually bring the pet in for someone else—often their aging parent (who is attached to the dog), so they're there out of obligation. Apathetic clients usually tell you right up front that they're only there because they have to be.

Apathetic clients' goal is to endure this obligatory trip to the vet and move on to the more important aspects of their day. Don't give them the bare minimum they ask for and then move on with your day. The pet deserves more than that. Apathetic clients need to hear a call to action.

You need to prod them into seeing the importance of the problem at hand. Apathetic clients are not there because of their relationship with the pet but because of their relationship with the pet's owner. Let them know that the recommended tests or treatments are geared to enhance the pet's life and therefore, by extension, the owner's life, too.

Victim

These poor pet owners are hapless victims of circumstance. They aren't happy about being at the veterinary clinic, and didn't want the pet anyway. Perhaps the pet was their child's before he or she went off to college, or their deceased parents', or just wandered into the front yard.

Victims' goal is to get out of the veterinary clinic after doing the bare minimum. Of course, they came into the clinic on their own, which suggests they have some bond with the animal. Don't pressure victims in any way. They don't want to say yes to anything, so don't put them in a yes-or-no position. Go through your normal physical exam process and narrate the problems that are present. At the end of the exam, highlight again what you've found. Most victims will then ask you what needs to be done, which gives you the opening you need to discuss the desired tests or treatments and the value of the various outcomes. If victims don't ask about the physical exam findings, then you'll need to move forward and discuss them anyway.

Victims want specifics and details. Whether they say it out loud or not, victims are doing the math while you're talking and calculating the cost:benefit ratio. Make certain you express the benefits and the future cost savings clearly—you may feel like a used car salesman, but doing this provides the information victims need. It's worth the effort because it's tough to predict what victims will decide—some do the math and decide to go for a $1,000 diagnostic and treatment plan, and others won't pay for more than the OFFICE call. Enough say yes to make it worth your while.

Conclusion

Hawks see their world as a construct of concrete and tangible facts. They're logical decision makers, so they'll spend more time discussing benefits and costs than asking how their pet will feel after treatment. Of course they care about their pet; they just express that caring in a different way than other cognitive styles.

Hawks are no-nonsense and don't appreciate hype, drama, or exaggeration. Because they're so straightforward, it's important to present information to them in a brief and sequential fashion.

CHAPTER 8

The Dog

Thump-thump-thump—the dog's tail wags as soon as you enter the room. He's just happy being part of the group and wants the group to be happy with him! Any adventure is okay—a walk around the block, a ride in the car—as long as he gets to participate.

Dogs at a Glance

Driving Force: Interaction, Relationships, Support, and Practicality

Dogs are all about relationships. Dogs feel validated and real by interacting with others—be it their pet, you, friends, or family.

Motto: "I Wanna Be Loved by You"

Dogs need to feel a personal connection with you. They don't want a cookie-cutter approach, and they want you to have enough time in the exam room so they can enjoy your company. In many cases, the most important relationship in their life is the one they have with their pet. Suggesting that they're being neglectful or hurtful will drive a wedge in that bond, and they may choose to shoot the messenger rather than listen to your advice.

Conversation Style: Fact-Based and Sequential but Potentially Clouded by Denial

Dogs want to preserve their relationships above all else. How these clients act in the exam room is based on whom that relationship is with. For example, many Dog owners will fail to administer medications as directed because the pet "doesn't like it" or "gets mad" at them.

Need Information to Be: Practical, Sequential, Empathetic, with Real-Life Examples

Dogs need objective information to make their decisions, but then somewhat paradoxically, they may seem to make those decisions on the basis of how it will affect those around them. They want to hear how other owners have addressed the issue.

Want to Know: What's Wrong and How Have Others Fixed It? What's to Be Gained by a Course of Action? How Will It Inconvenience the Pet and Them?

Dogs are the clients most likely to engage in full-blown denial. They would rather not know the truth than hear bad news. In some cases, their spouse has made an ultimatum that if the pet has an expensive problem, then it will have to be euthanized. So to a Dog, information can be a double-edged sword.

These clients will often refuse tests because they don't want to make the pet uncomfortable. A series of tests that takes all day or the prospect of the tests causing pain may make the Dog say no. It's not enough to explain the benefits—you need to show Dogs where the pet is kept and walked and make them realize that you'll attend to its comfort.

Become Angry When: They Perceive That You're Criticizing Their Care of the Pet or Don't Feel That You've Addressed Them Personally.

Dogs are grounded in the world of real facts but maintain a warm and fuzzy side. To succeed with them, you need to present the data without seeming cold and clinical.

Dogs are sensory-based—they can see that their pet is overweight. However, they react strongly to criticism, so it's best to gently point out the problems that need to be corrected, unless they ask you point-blank. (However, it's usually the Hawk in the room that asks the blunt question, so that the Dog can hear the answer—this is definitely the time to be tactful.)

After carefully pointing out a flaw or problem, you should quickly follow up with three pieces of information: (1) how the owner can make the necessary correction, (2) how the pet's life will be improved, and (3) real-life examples of pets you've known that benefited from the course of action.

Serious Medical Problems

Dogs are devastated by serious medical problems, because they realize that their relationship with the pet may be forever altered. Here again, it's important to present the facts, but in a supportive, empathetic fashion. Dogs don't want to be patronized or have things sugarcoated, but if you must be blunt, apologize for doing so in advance. They want help, and they need to know that you want to help them.

Emergencies

There's likely to be a lot of drama when Dogs have a pet with an emergency. In the absence of data, their mind is running wild with worst-case scenarios. It's up to you to throw them a life preserver in the form of some information that they can hold on to, emphasizing whatever positives you can find as you deliver the prognosis.

Dogs tend to be forgiving if an initially optimistic prognosis changes with more information. Of course, they'd rather hear only good news, but if you must deliver bad news, do so as kindly as possible.

Money

Most Dogs will do anything to preserve their relationship with the pet. They may be the classic owners who say, "Do whatever you need to," without giving any thought to the actual cost or how they'll pay. A prudent veterinarian will politely make certain that Dogs can pay for the authorized services.

Euthanasia and Grief

Most Dogs won't enter into the decision to euthanize lightly. You can expect the situation to be an emotional roller coaster. Dogs will definitely ask you, "Isn't there anything else that can be done?" and "What would you do if it was your pet?"

The Difficult Client

When you have difficulty with Dogs as clients, it's usually because they're trying to preserve the relationship with their pet, even when it no longer makes sense for the animal. This may make you feel like judge, jury, and executioner when the pet has run out of reasonable treatment options.

In some cases, the owner wants treatment for the pet but can't afford it and may pressure you to help him or her. Many veterinarians already do a lot of charity work. You have the right to make a living, so simply explain that the clinic can't afford to discount the cost of treatment. With their fact-oriented cognitive style, Dogs will understand this on some level. It is important not to make your end of the conversation emotionally charged, because it is the angry owner who is the most likely to report you to the licensing board.

If you're being tested by a Dog, it means the following:

- The Dog has interpreted something you said as a criticism of how he or she cares for the pet. Because the pet is usually their primary concern, Dogs view criticism as tantamount to calling them a pet abuser. Reassess your delivery and try to frame criticism in the form of a suggestion—for example, how a change will help the pet feel better and live longer.

- You have not established that you care about the pet or the owner. Perhaps you seem emotionally detached, too busy to listen, or as though you've made a diagnosis before you've even walked into the room.

- The Dog doesn't like people to stand on their soapbox. There are times when you have to say what you think, but emphasize the benefits of your proposal rather than focus on the negatives of some other treatment plan (e.g., an unproven herbal remedy that the Dog found on the Internet). Dogs receive positive messages better than they do negative ones.

Special Considerations with Social-Cognitive Style Combinations
Leader Dogs

Exuberant, funny, and friendly, Leader Dogs light up the exam room. They may get so focused on interacting with you that they forget the pet's problems, so after a couple of minutes of chatting, try to maintain the focus on the pet.

Leader Dogs are used to making decisions and being in charge—until there's conflict. Then they can quickly become hurt or defensive. Leader Dogs try to live up to others' expectations and want you to do the same. They are accommodating by nature, so try to clarify what it is they want or need from you so there aren't any misunderstandings.[163]

Energizer Dogs

Even though Energizer Dogs are fact-oriented, the talkative ones actually learn better by doing. Energizer Dogs won't absorb much from a handout or video about how to give an injection or clean the ears, but if you show them how to do it, they'll learn quickly and thank you for taking the time.

Energizer Dogs are always engaging, which means they will probably do 90 percent of the talking in the exam room. Their hyperactivity can make them seem flighty or unfocused, but they're usually very responsive when asked to do something (e.g., give the pet its medication). Energizer Dogs do live in the moment, so you may need to clearly explain the long-term consequences of a problem for them to understand its importance.

Engineer Dogs

Engineer Dogs are the type of client who will bring in a color-coded three-month journal of the dog's vomiting patterns. Take the time to look at the journal, and be sure to put a copy of it in the file. It'll help them feel respected and worthwhile.

Engineer Dogs have a tendency to develop a martyr complex or to be taken advantage of by others because they're sensitive to everyone else's needs and work diligently to satisfy them.[162] They also have a high sense of order and rules and will react negatively if they feel that you're cutting corners or not giving them all they expected. As Engineers, they are very detail-oriented, so they're going to want specifics on treatment and tests, not just the big picture.

Dreamer Dogs

These quiet, friendly pet owners are very sensitive. They seek harmony, acceptance, and a feeling of community. Support Dreamer Dogs and they'll support you. You should approach all conversations with them as though you are on the same team, although this approach can be challenging because Dreamer Dogs tend to have terrible follow-through and are unlikely to come back for recheck appointments or even give medication as directed. They aren't willfully defying your recommendations, though—they're just going in too many different directions to follow any of them.

Some Dogs You May Meet
Parent

The parent is an easy-to-identify client type. Parents will have the pet swaddled in their protective arms. For these owners, the relationship with the pet is the beginning and end of every day—and everything in between. Their pets are often overweight because parents can't bear to see the pet "not eat." The pet's pleasure is parents' main goal, and its pain is their main worry. Don't criticize the pet's care. Instead, try to be tactful, and talk about how some dogs can develop arthritis if they don't get enough exercise or get too much to eat. It may seem as if you're speaking in code, but this strategy prevents parents' defenses from coming up and their ears from closing.

When making recommendations, try to emphasize the pet's perspective. For example, you can say, "Those red gums mean that your pet's mouth is infected and probably painful. A dental cleaning will help, and then we can talk about strategies to prevent this from happening in the future." Deliver bad news to parents after you've given a complete exam. Parent owners are often overly sensitive and will stop listening if they hear negativity early in the process.

If parent owners say no, it may be because you haven't communicated the value of the treatment or test clearly enough. Remember, though, that parent owners don't assess benefits and costs the way most others do. They would rather chew off their own arm to avoid inconveniencing or harming the dog. Recognize that parent owners don't want to be separated from their animal for any amount of time, so even a two-hour test may seem like an eternity. Paint a picture of the care their beloved pet will receive while in the clinic: Show them where you walk the dogs when they stay at the clinic, tell them to bring the dog's favorite blanket and toy, and introduce them to some of the happy critters that are already there.

Brick Wall

Some clients are like brick walls—you just can't seem to get through to them. No matter what you say, there doesn't seem to be a way to elicit a response. You've had those exams during which the client barely made eye contact and never asked a question—you can't help but feel that an opportunity was lost in those cases. However, in a busy clinical setting, most veterinarians just shrug and move on to the next exam room.

You really do need to help these clients, because most of the time brick walls are terrified. They fear that something is terribly wrong with their pet, and they can't bear to face it. Brick walls are in see-no-evil, speak-no-evil, hear-no-evil mode. Their pet's problem has overstimulated them to the point of catatonia, and they've shut down. In many cases, brick walls are hypersensitive because of a previous experience at another veterinary clinic, or with another pet, or even with an ailing human family member.

Brick walls' goal is to make the scary situation go away and go back to how things were before the pet got sick. Don't aggravate the situation by getting frustrated if they're unresponsive or by becoming matter-of-fact. Don't overload them with details—they're not functioning at that level right now. When making recommendations, first and foremost find out what the real problem is. Terrified brick walls need comfort and reassurance. It may take some time to understand what the root of the problem is. In some cases, it may be a past negative experience; in others, it may be money ("I'm going to have to euthanize the pet if this costs too much"); and in others it's that the pet's problem mirrors that of a deceased love one. Once you understand what has caused them to become a brick wall, you can disassemble it brick by brick.

Brick walls feel powerless and like victims of circumstance. Give them the power and ability to make decisions. As they emerge from the fog of fear, you can give them more specific information about the pet's problems, but don't overdo it.

Rescuer

Here comes the rescuer—again—with yet another pet. These folks derive their sense of self and status from all of the pets they save. Some rescuers take great care of their foundlings, and others don't.

"Bad" rescuers are those people who have too many pets and too few resources to care for any of them adequately. They have a martyr complex and think it's up to them to save all these helpless pets that just keep showing up on their doorstep. Rescuers love saving the abused animal, and all of their pets have a hard-luck story. What's truly sad is that many of these rescuers actually lack healthy relationships with other people, so they create a not-always-healthy relationship with their rescued animals. To rescuers, each pet is another stone in the foundation of their self-image. The more stones there are, the stronger the foundation. Rescuers' goals are to (1) enhance their self-image by bringing the pet to you, (2) have you compliment them on their caring and kindness, and (3) help the pet.

Although it may be difficult, try not to overtly criticize the pet's condition. Rescuers have often bitten off more than they can chew and may honestly not be able to afford to care for their animals. However, you can't condone substandard or neglectful care, so discussing the pet's needs may require some diplomacy. When making recommendations, acknowledge how hard it can be to take good care of a pet. List the problems that you see with this animal (write them down) and the remedies for those problems, and prioritize them. The list may be long, and euthanasia may be one of the proposed remedies. Finally, list the costs of the proposed treatment plans.

> *To rescuers, each pet is another stone in the foundation of their self-image. The more stones there are, the stronger the foundation.*

Bad rescuers have issues that go beyond codependency with pets and substandard care, and they'll process your information very slowly. Recognize that euthanizing a pet gives rescuers one less stone in the foundation of their self-image, so an animal's death is more than the loss of a pet, it is also a loss of a piece of their identity.

Find a way to enhance rescuers' self-image by emphasizing how much better the pet will feel if treated; how they can learn from this disease to better care for their other pets; or, if euthanasia is the answer, even though this pet will be missed, they'll have more time to take care of the other pets that are so special to them.

Conclusion

Dogs are sensory-driven and fact-based but have a softer, more emotional side. Relationships are very important to Dogs, so they'll work hard to maintain their connection to their pet as well as to their veterinarian. Dogs' feelings can easily get hurt if they feel that you're criticizing the care they give their pet, and they'll become angry if they feel you're threatening that relationship.

Dog owners appreciate anecdotes about other cases that you've seen and how other owners have handled the same situation. Although they want facts, quoting a textbook isn't going to satisfy Dogs. They don't want to be treated like a number. Value and respect Dogs' relationship with their pet, and they'll be loyal clients.

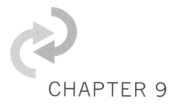

CHAPTER 9

The Kitten

The kitten jumps in the air, races across the couch, climbs up the wall, and then plops down under a chair (all in the span of five seconds). It may or may not do it again— not even the kitten seems to know what direction it's headed in next. For the kitten, having a direction isn't the point; it's enjoying life that's so important.

Kittens at a Glance
Driving Force: Individuality, Creativity, Ongoing Growth, Acceptance of Other People's Values

Kittens are likeable and want to be liked in kind. They don't push their values on you, and ask that you accept theirs as well. Kittens are creative and are often free spirits. They'll think outside the box and expect you to respect their relationships with their pet.

Motto: "Live and Let Live"

Kittens want to be appreciated for who they are. Their carefree approach to life has received criticism from others and that turns them off, because they aren't naturally critical. For these clients, the journey of life is more important than the destination. Therefore, quality of life is the most important consideration for their pet.

Conversation Style: Interactive, Friendly, Easygoing, and Respectful

Kittens are looking for a broad understanding of their pet's problems. They'll share their observations with you—even those that are clearly not relevant. They want to make certain that you have all the information. Kittens want to connect with you on a personal level and will appreciate time taken to get to know them.

Need Information to Be: Noncritical, Kind-Hearted, Sincere, Considerate of All Options and Who Will Be Affected

Kittens' creative and spontaneous side may make them seem scattered. Kittens aren't usually linear thinkers, so they aren't connecting data points to make their decisions. Instead, they need a clear idea of how a decision will affect their quality of life as well as that of their pet. They're very genuine people, and they want you to interact with them on a similar level; they value honesty and kindness.

Want to Know: What Is Wrong with Their Pet? How Will It Affect All Involved? What Are Some Other Options?

Kittens are all about their pet's fun. Although they're not as permissive as Dogs, they aren't likely to have very well-behaved pets, either.

Kittens want to talk about all of the holistic therapies and need to know that you've considered them as well. If you simply slam the door on alternative treatments, you'll seem unfairly critical to them. Instead, talk about your experience with these products—mention a few specific cases and how the pet was helped or not helped by holistic treatments. Kittens will accept this information more readily than any scientific paper you can quote.

Because Kittens are all about the journey, they want to know that their pet is having fun every day. They can accept short-term inconvenience (confinement for a month after fracture repair) for long-term gain, but they don't handle the concept of chronic pain very well.

Become Angry When: You Suggest Their Pet's Health Problem Is Their Fault

Kittens are doing the best they can for their animal, and if they have contributed to their pet's health problem, then it's unintentional. Criticism and a lack of mutual respect are real issues for a Kitten. Kittens need to feel that you have the time to see them and talk with them as individuals. This doesn't necessarily translate into a 50-minute OFFICE call; they just have to feel that you're unhurried and focused on them. If you're preoccupied, interrupted frequently during the OFFICE call, or otherwise seem distracted, then they'll be unhappy clients.

These owners don't just think outside the box; sometimes they think off the planet. Many of their thoughts may seem absurd, but Kittens occasionally have a moment of insight or brilliance that you haven't considered. If they want to pursue an alternative modality that won't hurt their pet, then don't discourage it. Dismissing their questions won't win you any friends. Kittens don't accept an authoritarian model of medical care; they instead need you to be an encouraging coach.

Serious Medical Problems

Kittens may seem a little less worried than they should be about serious health problems. They innately think there are other options that haven't been considered, so even a grave prognosis is not an absolute to them. Fortunately, this doesn't manifest as denial. Kittens seem to float on the sea of life, and they accept that sometimes the current takes them in a different direction than they'd hoped.

When breaking bad news to Kittens, it's important that they feel you've considered all the possibilities when making your diagnosis and prognosis. Deliver bad news kindly. Kittens are sensitive creatures, and they need empathy in tough situations.

Emergencies

Grace under pressure is likely to be the initial reaction of the Kitten in an emergency situation. They're used to things just happening in their life, because Kittens aren't great planners and don't schedule their own lives. Although an emergency is unexpected, so is everything else that happens to them.

Give Kittens some initial positive feedback in an emergency situation, and they'll take a deep breath and let you go to work. Of course, they want everything to work out well for their suddenly injured or ill animal, but Kittens have the most adaptable cognitive style if the pet takes a turn for the worse. Keep Kittens in the loop, let them know all the efforts you're making and problems you're treating, and they'll be satisfied that you're doing a good job.

Money

Kittens aren't as concerned about the money as they are about the pet's quality of life. Not known for being great accountants, Kittens may be tempted to authorize expensive treatment that they can't afford, as long as you say the pet is going to be fine.

This situation can be tricky, because you can end up taking advantage of a Kitten unintentionally. They do mean to pay but may not have the ability to do so, so you may have to put the brakes on a treatment plan and explain that you need to qualify them for a payment plan, make a deposit, or otherwise follow your client payment policy.

Euthanasia and Grief

Euthanasia is always a tough decision, but Kittens seem to be in tune with their pet's quality of life. When they've reached the decision that euthanasia is the best choice, it's after some lengthy internal deliberation.

Most Kittens will want to talk with you about the process by which they made the decision—how the dog can no longer stand on the kitchen floor, the time they found it in a puddle of urine, and so forth. Being noncritical by nature, they aren' t comfortable making these types of decisions, and they'll be thankful that you've listened and explained that euthanasia may be the kindest, most humane option.

The Difficult Client

When Kittens get mad at you, it means that they don't feel you respected their personal or specific issues. Perhaps you seemed too hurried or appeared to make the diagnosis before hearing all of the information. Even if you made the correct diagnosis, they still want their unique observations to be noted and considered.

Special Considerations with Social-Cognitive Style Combinations
Leader Kittens

These outgoing and intuitive folks are very in tune with your mood and the clinic's interpersonal environment. If they're unhappy, it may be that they've picked up on workplace tension and are concerned that it will affect the care their pet receives. They'll take advice that sounds like criticism very personally.

Energizer Kittens

Naturally indecisive and gregarious Energizer Kittens will seem as though they're leaping all over the place in the exam room. They are easily influenced by outside forces and will give equal weight to your advice and their friends' input as well as that of some guy down the street. It can be a chore to keep them focused on the pet's problem and the steps to resolve it, and you'll need to listen to the other information they've learned to allow Kittens to feel that you're considering all the alternatives.

Engineer Kittens

Engineer Kittens are classic scholars, and as such they can have a tendency to over-analyze a situation or complicate even the simplest problem. They're very sensitive to criticism, but because they're reserved, you'll likely never know that you've somehow offended them.

Dreamer Kittens

The most idealistic of the Kittens (which is the most idealistic of the four cognitive styles), Dreamer Kittens may seem as though they have their heads in the clouds. They will ignore a pet's problem—not through denial, but because they think that things are likely to get better on their own. They're extremely troubled by conflict, so it's important to make certain that you stay on the same team as they are no matter what the pet's problem is.

Some Kittens You May Meet
Know-It-All

These Kittens know everything. Know-it-alls may even try to finish your sentences for you, and they're typically worse if there's an audience in the exam room. Let them talk—they're going to anyway. When they pause to take a breath, say, "That's an excellent point," and then go on with what you were trying to say.

Know-it-alls are the self-appointed experts in the family, and now they're on your turf. Visualize the nervous Chihuahua that barks and lunges at bigger dogs during a walk, and you have a good idea where these folks are mentally. It's not that they intend to be domineering; they just live in a self-constructed world, and you threaten to burst their bubble. Don't try to challenge or educate this client directly.

When making recommendations, try to build on know-it-alls' knowledge and then redirect them in a more constructive direction. Rephrasing what know-it-alls say and incorporating it into the information you provide will guarantee that they're listening, because the only thing they like better than hearing themselves talk is hearing their words repeated.

If know-it-alls say no, don't spend a lot of time trying to pressure them. By saying no, they're once again in charge of the exam room. Instead, ask whether you can send home some information for them to consider, and then set up a time to call and talk with them directly about the proposed test or procedure. Don't say, "I'll call to answer your questions," because the know-it-all won't have any. Pick a particular time to call, and write it on the handout you send home.

Wonderers

Wonderers are always exploring—everything. They want all of the answers before they'll commit to anything, and they'll ask big-picture questions. Sometimes Wonderers like to throw a monkey wrench into the gears when they're asked to make a decision (e.g., "I can drop the pet off by 8:00 but can't pick it up at 3:00"). This monkey wrench is often just a way to buy time while Wonderers continue to explore the world around them.

With an endless litany of (not always pertinent) questions, they manifest "paralysis by analysis." After you've provided a thorough and exhaustive discussion of all the possible outcomes of a recommended test or procedure, Wonderers may still look at you blankly, waiting for more detail. You'll have to ask them whether they want to move forward or think about it.

Wonderers need only a superficial understanding of their pet's problem but a clear big-picture diagram of how to treat it. They need to know what will happen with and without treatment. Although Wonderers aren't happy that their pet is ill, in many cases the animal's illness has been made worse because they failed to act, hoping that everything would work out on its own. Wonderers are about hope, imagination, and their pet's lifestyle, and you need to talk with them on this level rather than try to persuade them with sterile scientific facts.

Don't overload the conversation with details, because details sound like "blah blah blah" to the Wonderer. Don't repeat yourself unless you're asked for clarification—Wonderers aren't dumb; they just don't color within the lines. Don't tell Wonderers what to do. They resist hype and pressure.

Storyteller

Everyone knows a storyteller. He or she may be the client or a friend of the client's who came along for support. Storytellers need an audience, so a trip to the vet is somewhat self-serving. By definition, storytellers are outgoing, and they usually talk rapidly and loudly. They may ask you what's wrong with their pet two seconds after you've entered the exam room. To keep them occupied during the physical exam, you might ask storytellers to tell you what's been going on. That's all the invitation the storyteller needs.

Storytellers like being the center of attention. Any encouragement you give—nodding your head, saying "uh-huh" or "wow"—will just add fuel to the fire. Maintain your focus on the pet. Storytellers love the process of interacting with you, especially if their pet can propel them onto center stage. The pet may seem like a prop, but they did bring it to you for a reason, so give them due credit.

Although you don't want storytellers to ramble needlessly, it's not necessary to interrupt them. You may feel like a captive, but you don't have to be captivated—just go through the physical exam and then regain eye contact with the storyteller when you're ready.

If storytellers are on a roll, you may need to find a polite way to interrupt them so that you can ask a question. A gesture to catch storytellers' attention may work (e.g., direct eye contact and a smile, raising your hand), and waiting for a lull and saying "excuse me" is often effective.

You probably shouldn't ask storytellers a lot of open-ended questions; instead, ask yes-or-no questions and hope you'll get through your list before new stories are told. These folks aren't very detail-oriented, so you'll have to ask for the specific information you need.

Storytellers are usually more big-picture people. Don't bore them with details about how arthritis medication will give their pet an increased range of motion; instead, tell them that their pet will walk more comfortably, be more willing to play, and generally be happier.

The Truth About Kittens and Dogs

In the clinical setting, Kittens and Dogs can be difficult to distinguish. Here are some scenarios to help you distinguish between the two types.

Scenario 1

A client comes in with an unruly dog. When you suggest obedience training, the client seems offended. Is this client a Kitten or a Dog?

Kittens will be offended by the notion of obedience training because they are free spirits. "He's fine at home" will be a Kitten's common response. They aren't put out by the notion of obedience training; they just don't see the point.

A Dog's dog won't be well trained because this owner doesn't want to be the bad person and enforce discipline. You may see a look of anguish on the Dog's face as he or she thinks about the last tantrum the dog had when disciplined. This owner will likely defend the dog ("He's never tried to bite before") or excuse the dog ("It's not his fault; he's just nervous here.")

Scenario 2

You examine an older dog that clearly has arthritis and recommend anti-inflammatory medication. The owner argues that the dog doesn't have arthritis. Is this client a Kitten or a Dog?

Dogs may engage in denial and not want to see that their pet is aging. These clients will argue that their pet must not have arthritis because it never cries in pain. Most Dogs project their own feelings onto their pet and expect the animal to behave as if it were a furry little person. Dogs need to see concrete evidence of the arthritis before they will believe that it is there.

If a Kitten's pet can still do the things that it likes to do—go for walks, chase a ball—then the Kitten will conclude that the pet must not have arthritis. Because the pet's quality of life doesn't seem to be adversely affected, the problem must not exist. For Kittens, the need for any ongoing treatment is going to be a value judgment based on the pet's happiness or well-being. (See Table 9.1.)

TABLE 9.1 The Truth About Kittens and Dogs

Information Gathering	Kittens	Dogs
Perception of time	Willing to think about tomorrow	Focused on the present
Perception of care	Take an "if it ain't broke, don't fix it" approach to pet care	Worry about the pet's feelings when there's a change (e.g., going on a diet)
Flexibility	Likely to explain why a change isn't necessary	Will be defensive personally or on behalf of the pet when a change is proposed

Conclusion

Kittens are fun-loving, intuitive, and free-spirited people. They enjoy their pets for what they are, and don't try to impose on them. People with this idealistic cognitive style tend to feel that everything is going to work out, which can make them slow at identifying a pet's health problem and seeking veterinary help. Veterinarians may find Kittens difficult to converse with at times because they are naturally abstract in their thinking, and it's difficult to bring them along a sequential train of thought.

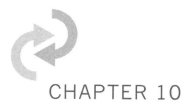

CHAPTER 10

The Owl

Sitting on a tree branch, the owl looks to the left, then the right. He looks up and down. The owl is a keen observer of all that goes on around him. With his insight, the owl strives to make sense of the world.

Owls at a Glance
Driving Force: Organization, Theoretical Understanding, Honesty, and Competence

Owls strive to understand the world at a deeper level than most. They're looking for patterns and formulas others don't notice. They challenge standard dogma and spend most of their time thinking outside the box.

Although intuitive by nature, Owls are almost scientific in their thought processes and want information presented in an organized and comprehensible framework. They'll do the free thinking from there.

Motto: "I Think, Therefore I Am"

Owls are problem solvers and long-range planners. In fact, they may spend more time talking about the various outcomes of a treatment plan than about its day-to-day implementation. Again, this can be good and bad—an Owl may focus on the long-term negative side effects of nonsteroidal anti-inflammatory drugs and ignore the immediate benefits of arthritis relief.

Conversation Style: Theoretical, Skeptical, and Analytical

Owls want information, but not necessarily data. They'll ask for the why and how behind the data. From there, Owls will try tp reprogram the information and make it their own. Sometimes this may come across as ingenious; sometimes it may appear that they doubt your conclusions. Owls don't intend to criticize you or your knowledge; this is simply the Owl's process.

Need Information to Be: Organized, Balanced, Logical, and Prospective

Owls reject conventional knowledge when coming up with their own worldview. They'll listen respectfully to you but then ask specific follow-up questions to challenge why you think the way you do. Owls are looking for you to provide a scaffold of information so that they can start to theorize on their own. Owls understand that all actions have good and bad consequences, and they want both sides presented fairly and logically.

These clients are always thinking about the future, and they can sometimes "fly away" on too much future-think. Owls want to go on a journey of understanding, and they may want to find out what will happen at every single fork in the road.

Want to Know: What's the Current Problem? What Are the Possible Explanations? What Tests Need to Be Run to Filter the Results? What Are the Implications of All Treatment Plans?

Insightful and analytical, Owls quickly grasp the key points when you're explaining their pet's health problem. However, their questions quickly move beyond basic understanding and into the realm of theory. You may find this frustrating because veterinarians are used to getting clients to the level of basic understanding and no further. That's not enough for Owls!

Owls will question every possible diagnostic and treatment plan—not to challenge you (although it may feel that way), but instead to gain greater insight. Try to provide Owls with a good framework of information, present the pros and cons of all treatment plans, and then supplement this information with links to quality websites for their own research. Invite Owls to look at the information and then call back with questions so you can discuss it further. They seldom call back, but if they do, their questions and insights are often interesting enough to make it worth your while.

Become Angry When: You Say "Because That's the Way It Is" and Haven't Seemed to Consider the Possibilities.

Owls don't want you to tell them anything; they'd rather come to their own conclusions. Owls will grow frustrated if you present information in a random and disorganized fashion. They're logical thinkers, and they'll respect you for your sequential, organized delivery. Owls need options—they want to sort the information and make their own choices, so give them enough detail to help them make the best choices for their pet.

Serious Medical Problems

Serious medical problems frustrate Owls because they feel the world should be organized and systematic—and emergencies fall outside of their schedule. Owls will want to consider all possible explanations for the pet's condition and then ponder all possible outcomes.

In the early stages of a pet's serious medical problem, try to stay light on the details. For example, a vomiting dog may have raided the garbage can, been poisoned, swallowed a toy, have Addison's disease, or numerous other possibilities. If you introduce all the differentials, be prepared to speak in depth about each one of them.

The challenge is to provide Owls with sufficient information without trapping yourself in an endless loop of explanation, but that's exactly what you need to do. In the case of a vomiting dog, you might suggest three possibilities (e.g., the dog ate something rotten, has a hormonal imbalance, or has an infection) and then explain how you're going to determine the cause. If the answer is different from your proposed differentials, an Owl will be okay with that, so long as you've come up with the right answer. The Owl may then become interested (and excited!) in why you ran that particular test and how you figured out what the real problem was.

Emergencies

By definition, emergencies are random and unexpected, and they upset the Owl's need for patterns, predictability, and understanding. In the emergency setting, Owls want you to give them a game plan from the beginning. They want to hear about the possibilities in a broad sense and how the emergency is going to affect the pet in the long term. Owls can accept that you don't have all the answers immediately, but they need to know how you'll systematically get the answers. They want the information as you get it, so it's important to keep them up to speed and allow them to process, filter, and ask questions as you work through the emergency. Respect an Owl's intelligence and need for information, and you'll have a satisfied client.

Money

Owls tend to be practical about money. They want to know that there's valuable information to be gained by the diagnostic tests that you want to run and need to understand why you want to run a particular test. Owls are very comfortable with broad, general tests—a standard chemistry panel—but they may balk when you want to run an expensive test that looks for just one thing. Be prepared to explain why a specific test is necessary. Owls are analytical by nature, and they'll want to know what will happen if they don't okay a test, so you need to explain how the results of a test may influence the treatment plan or potentially impair the pet's recovery.

Euthanasia and Grief

Because Owls are future-focused, they tend to grasp quickly when their pet's quality of life has become seriously compromised. Once their pet has shown a consistent trend of decline, Owls will make the decision to euthanize, and they'll appreciate your reassurance when they've made this tough decision. Owls don't typically euthanize a pet too soon, but if you think they're making this decision prematurely, then you need to first listen to all of their observations before introducing other alternatives.

The Difficult Client

The biggest difficulty with Owls is that they have an insatiable need for knowledge. They'll respect you if you provide understandable information and become angry or difficult if you (1) talk over their head, (2) don't provide them with alternatives, (3) don't focus on the long term, or (4) add hype or melodrama to the situation.

Special Considerations with Social-Cognitive Style Combinations
Leader Owl

Leader Owls are outgoing strategists, and they'll look at their pet's problem as a puzzle that needs to be solved. They won't be satisfied unless you find an explanation for their pet's problem—for example, even if your treatment plan has resolved their pet's significant gastroenteritis, they won't feel that you've done your job properly unless you find the cause.

Leader Owls have a tendency to come across as overly intellectual, which you may find intimidating or annoying. Leader Owls aren't trying to outthink you, but they can be more insightful than most folks around them, which can make them seem arrogant at times. Enlist the Leader Owl as a codetective in solving the "Case of the Pet's Problem," and you'll have an ally throughout the process.

Energizer Owl

Dynamic Energizer Owls are competitive and supportive at the same time. Nothing is ever final for this indecisive personality type, so they'll agree with your diagnostic plan one minute and then argue against it the next. They can seem very similar to Kittens (most specifically Energizer Kittens) because both are outgoing and abstract thinkers, but Owls will be more focused on future consequences and Kittens usually just want to return the pet to its previous healthy state.

Engineer Owl

Engineer Owls are the most independent thinkers of all personality types—which can be good and bad. It can be good because they're usually pretty smart, and bad because they don't ever stop trying to tinker with a problem or situation. Engineer Owls are likely to have researched the dose and frequency of a medication you've prescribed and ask why you're administering it one way instead of another. This strategy doesn't make them seem like much of a team player, and in fact, they're not. Engineer Owls are used to being in charge of their own little corner of the world. When they come into your clinic, they have a difficult time allowing you to take charge.

Dreamer Owl

The Dreamer Owl may be a wolf in sheep's clothing. These folks have usually done their homework before they've come into the exam room and will ask very specific and relevant questions from the start. They're easygoing but on an endless quest for knowledge. What you may find challenging is that Dreamer Owls never feel as though they have enough information, so if you allow it, they may keep you in the exam room asking questions. Give Dreamer Owls the big picture, and then direct them to some resources to fill in the blanks on their own. Dreamer Owls may have a hard time coming to a decision, so you'll need to frame the options carefully and let them know that it's time to make a choice.

Some Owls You May Meet
Professor (Also Known as the Doubting Thomas)

Professors are deep thinkers. They want to know everything about everything, and they may remind you of the three-year-old who keeps asking why no matter what you say. Professors are intellectuals who love learning new things. They may be clever and remember what you say later, or they may just want to probe the depths of your knowledge. Don't tell professors that they won't understand something if you explain it to them. They want you to teach them—so teach.

When making recommendations, remember that professors want to visit every part of the forest before deciding on a diagnostic or treatment plan. The trick is to introduce them to a couple of the most important trees in the forest and focus on those. Your task is to provide enough information so that professors leave with more knowledge than when they started—without taking the time to give them a complete overview of every possibility.

Try to be as organized and systematic in your delivery as possible. Give a concise explanation of the advantages and disadvantages of your recommendations. Give the reasonable options. Use a dry-erase board for clarity. Professors want balance, so give them both sides.

Professors need time to process and arrive at their own decision—they're looking for the alternative that you haven't considered yet. Professors aren't decisive people—they're always leaving the door open for more information and new ideas, which makes it difficult for them to choose a specific course of action. Ask whether you can provide any more information to help them, and then leave them to process the information. Recommend a follow-up exam a few days later to give them a timeline for a decision.

There are three main reasons why professors may say no to a reasonable plan: (1) Even with your explanation, they don't understand or believe the need for it; (2) they want to analyze the situation further and come to their own conclusions; and (3) they're so analytical that they can't make any decision.

With professor Owls, you may have to conclude the explanatory phase and ask them point-blank whether you can run a specific test. Some are so theoretical they have a difficult time giving you a simple yes-or-no answer—because nothing is that simple in their world. Explain to them that the test will allow you to know which part of the forest you're in, so that you can clearly navigate a path toward the pet's well-being.

Litigator

It may seem as though litigators just want an argument. It's not clear whether they're trying to impress someone or just like playing devil's advocate. Litigators are almost always men.[158] Litigators wait for you to say something and then pounce on it.

Litigators are extroverts who want your full attention, not a cookie-cutter approach to medicine. To make certain you're individualizing your recommendations for their pet, they'll ask questions that seem to focus on the "why should I" of a particular test or treatment, not on what will be gained. If you aren't careful, they may let you talk yourself into a corner. Litigators' questions may just as likely be a test to see whether you believe in yourself. Don't get frustrated and adopt a "because I'm the doctor" attitude. Most litigators become great clients; they just have to put you through the gauntlet the first time to see if you have the "right stuff."

When making recommendations, try to focus on the net gain to litigator Owls personally as well as to their pet. They want facts and details, but they need to know that you see the big picture. For example, they may know that arthritis medicine may mean their pet will live a longer life with fewer other health problems (e.g., urinary tract infections, inability to go outside without help); however, they'll also want to discuss the long-term side effects of arthritis medicine. Litigator Owls will want to know how often the medication will need to be given, what happens if a dose is skipped, how expensive it will be, and so forth. In other words, litigators want to know how treatment will help their pet but also how it will inconvenience everyone else. Once you've passed their tests, litigators can become your biggest and most vocal fans.

Worrier

The expression on this Owl's face will let you know the moment you walk into the exam room that you're dealing with a worrier. At first, you may think this client is an overprotective or concerned parent type, but parents' questions will deal with their pet's feelings (happy, painful, etc.); worriers will acknowledge those feelings but want to understand the big picture of their pet's condition.

Worriers' goal is to eliminate uncertainty. Worriers live an organized and rational life. When their pet has a specific problem, this reality upsets Worriers' theoretically stable world. This client needs information to be provided in an organized, straightforward, and balanced framework.

Worriers share some of their world outlook with Wonderers, but they're more black-and-white when putting a plan into action. Worriers can come to a decision once they have all of the information, so getting them that information is the key. Worriers don't need hype or drama to recognize the severity of their pet's issues. Providing too much detail, at least initially, can be a hindrance, because worriers may want to know more about how the data were derived than about what they actually mean.

When making recommendations, paint a big picture of the pet's problem, and then slowly fill in the details, based on the owner's questions. Worriers want to know about possibilities and alternatives, and they also want to know about the future outcomes. They'll actually read your handouts carefully, so make sure they say what you want them to say. Recommend websites that have good information. Worriers may ask about experimental or holistic treatments, but they're

TABLE 10.1   Client Cognitive Types

At a Glance	Hawks	Dogs	Kittens	Owls
Driving force	Efficiency, accountability, benefit	Interaction, relationships, support	Individuality, ongoing growth, relationships	Organization, theory, competence
Communication style	Straightforward, based on observable fact	Emphasizes feelings, quality of life	Easygoing, interactive, meandering	Analytical, theoretical, skeptical
Needs information to be	Brief, relevant, sequential, unbiased	Practical, based on real-life experience, empathetic	Noncritical, kind-hearted, sincere	Organized, balanced, logical
Wants to know	What, how, and how much	Who is affected? What have others done?	What's wrong and how will it affect the pet's lifestyle?	Everything past, present, and especially future
Becomes angry when	Costs exceed estimates; unforeseen complications occur	You seem uncaring; life-or-death decisions	You imply that they've harmed their pet	Information seems biased, emotional, or one-sided
Money	Is always part of the equation	Will preserve the relationship at any cost	Don't care about money, but may not have any	Tend to be practical
Emergencies	Don't handle unknown very well	Acknowledge emotions before delivering facts	May seem calm but are still functioning on an emotional level	Need to know the game plan to bring order to chaos
Euthanasia	May seem cold, uncaring	Much angst before making decision	Will want to talk about making the right decision	Has a good sense of pet's quality of life
Becomes difficult when	Questions aren't being answered	Feel that they don't have any choices	Feel you're imposing your value system on them	Double-talk, hype, or melodrama occurs

generally grounded in the known world. There's no reason to be defensive; worrier Owls just want to explore all the options before settling on a course of therapy.

Conclusion

Owls are deep thinkers and problem solvers; however, they tend to be thinking about tomorrow's problems and can have a difficult time focusing on the issue at hand. They're both intuitive and logical, which creates an interesting cognitive blend, because they don't need data to fuel their stepwise and sequential thought processes. Owls are future-focused, and clients who are always asking about the repercussions of a treatment are likely Owls.

Table 10.1 displays the client cognitive types at a glance. Do you recognize any of your clients in the descriptions?

CHAPTER 11

Conversing with All Cognitive Styles via the FALE System

By now it should be clear that different personality types want and need different kinds of information. Identifying your clients as Hawks, Dogs, Kittens, or Owls will allow you to converse with them in the best way possible for their cognitive style: Hawks want to know the bottom line, Dogs wonder how a problem will affect their relationship with the pet, Kittens want the freedom to live and let live, and Owls need to understand the big picture.

This book has given you some tools for determining clients' various cognitive styles and communicating with them. But how do you converse effectively with clients when you can't quickly identify which cognitive style they have? What if several cognitive style types are present in the exam room?

The good news is that the FALE system—facts, alternatives, logic, and empathy—will allow you to communicate with all your clients, regardless of type.[42,161,163] Wait to deploy the FALE system until you're ready to talk—after the introductions have been made, the pet's been examined, and you've begun to develop a list of problems. Start by communicating the following:

- *Facts:* What the client has told you and what you've observed
- *Alternatives:* What the possible problems are, an overview of the different tests, and the various routes to try to home in on the problem
- *Logic:* A structure or framework for the diagnostic or treatment plan
- *Empathy:* Your concern for the pet and acknowledgment of how the pet's illness will affect the owner

    If you've provide FALE, you have communicated with all four cognitive styles:

- Hawks want facts and logic.
- Dogs need facts and empathy.
- Kittens hope for alternatives and empathy.
- Owls demand alternatives and logic.

    See Table 11.1.

TABLE 11.1 The FALE System Speaks to All Temperaments

Decision Making	Information Gathering	
	Facts	Alternatives
Logic	Hawk	Owl
Empathy	Dog	Kitten

FALE = facts, alternatives, logic, empathy

The FALE system works by conversing with each group via talking to *all* groups; it might sound time-consuming, but it's not.

Using the FALE System

Case Study 1

You've just examined a dog with a significant upset stomach. There could be stomach ulceration or it might lead to hemorrhagic gastroenteritis—it's too early to tell. As you start to explain the problem and suggest an overnight hospitalization, the owner asks, "Can't you just give him a shot, Doc?" Have you failed as a communicator? Definitely not; the key is to realize that each cognitive type will ask that question for a different reason: Hawks want an injection because they think it will be more efficient and cost-effective, Dogs wants a shot because it may mean their pet will feel better right away, and Kittens aren't convinced that the pet is so sick that it requires a night of hospitalization. Owls would never ask this question unless they wanted to discuss the various injections you might give and how they would interact with one another.

Using the FALE system, you'd explain the following:

- *Facts*: The pet has an irritated digestive tract and is dehydrated.
- *Alternatives*: The problem has several possible causes, and treatment is necessary to correct dehydration and heal the stomach (intravenous fluids, stomach protectants, antacids, etc.).
- *Logic*: Hospitalization is the best treatment plan.
- *Empathy*: My goal is to have your pet happy and at home as soon as possible. These treatments are the best way to accomplish that.

As you can see, no matter the owner's cognitive style, he will understand why "just giving a shot" won't solve the problem.

Case Study 2

You meet a new client who has brought her cat in for vaccines. You learn through listening and taking a history that the cat primarily lives indoors and only goes outside occasionally. You say, "I'd recommend three vaccines for your cat: feline distemper, leukemia, and rabies." The owner asks, "Why?" Your response might be, "Because it is clinic policy for cats that go outside to get all three vaccines." However, that answer may not have addressed the owner's actual question. *Why* has different meanings depending on whether the person asking is a Hawk, Dog, Kitten, or Owl.

When Hawks ask "why," they want to know the benefits versus the risks and whether they're getting their money's worth; Dogs are worried about vaccine reactions and whether the cat really needs to be poked three times; Kittens wonder whether the vaccines are necessary for their cat's lifestyle; and Owls need to understand how an appropriate vaccine protocol is determined. Unfortunately, your response didn't address the real question being asked by most cognitive styles.

Using the FALE system, you would explain the following:

- *Facts*: These three vaccines are generally the most important for indoor-outdoor cats.
- *Alternatives*: The vaccine protocol can always be modified for this specific cat.
- *Logic*: Occasionally, a cat may be attacked by or exposed to a sick stray cat, even in our own backyard. Also, the risk of a vaccine reaction is extremely low.
- *Empathy*: Three vaccines are likely to make the cat feel under the weather for part of the day, but by breakfast time tomorrow, it'll be back to its normal kitty behavior.

In my clinical experience, this explanation is more than enough to satisfy all cognitive types almost all of the time—the only exception is the owner who is highly sensitized to the possible dangers of overvaccinating (usually a Dog).

Case Study 3

You want to do preanesthetic bloodwork on an eight-year-old dog that is getting spayed. The client points out that the dog has had other surgeries without any problems, so why should he pay for expensive bloodwork now?

Using the FALE system, you respond with the following:

- *Facts:* As dogs age, the risk of anesthesia does increase. Although it's terrific that this dog hasn't had problems in the past, a number of issues can remain silent until you look for them.
- *Alternatives:* If you see a problem with the bloodwork, you can correct it before the surgery and reduce risk, tailor an anesthetic protocol to minimize the risk, or decide that the surgery is too risky and cancel it.

- *Logic:* Getting the dog spayed has benefits because it reduces the chance of uterine infections and mammary cancer. If the bloodwork looks good, it's better to do the surgery now than wait until the dog is even older.

- *Empathy:* You'll discuss the blood results with the client before doing anything and make certain that he is comfortable moving forward with surgery. If there's a problem, you'll work together to develop a plan to address it. The dog will definitely benefit from being spayed, and it likely will help her live a longer and happier life. Surgery is scary, but you and the client are making sure that it is the right thing for the dog and it will have the speediest recovery possible.

The Hawk has heard what he or she needs to feel that the bloodwork is worth the money—the dog will likely live longer and have fewer problems in the future. The Dog is relieved that bloodwork will make certain that the surgery is as safe as possible and that any problems it uncovers can be dealt with. The Kitten wants to make certain that all of the alternatives are considered because the dog isn't having any problems right now, but understands that surgery will probably result in the dog's having fewer health problems in the future. The Owl sees that the big picture of the dog's overall health is being considered and that there will be information from the bloodwork that will pinpoint potential issues down the road. All the cognitive types are satisfied, and it wasn't even that much work!

Conclusion

Hawks, Dogs, Kittens, and Owls vary in how they gather information and make decisions. The FALE system allows veterinarians to converse with all cognitive types at the same time, by giving each what he or she needs to be satisfied. This is particularly helpful if the client's cognitive style isn't obvious, or in the case in which multiple cognitive styles are present in the same exam room.

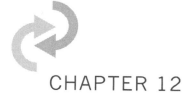

CHAPTER 12

Assessing Your Own Veterinary Conversation Style

If you're reading this book in sequence, then you've no doubt gained some insight into your own social-cognitive style combination. This insight will give you an idea about your preferred conversation style. Understanding your preferred style will help you to communicate more effectively, not only with clients, but in all facets of your life. Now you are ready for the "Personality Assessment" in Figure 12.1. Please take it now, and then we'll further explore your preferences. (This assessment also appears in Appendix A in case you want to make copies or take it more than once.)

Refer to Tables 12.1 and 12.2 for scoring procedures. If you scored a 5–6 or 6–5 on A + B, C + D, E + F, or G + H, then you have proven what complex creatures people are! If your scores are close, then explore the other cognitive-social style combination. Sometimes people's public personality is different from their private one, and this will show up on the test.

FIGURE 12.1   Personality Assessment

Are you a Leader Dog, a Dreamer Kitten, or somewhere in between?

In each group of two questions, circle the number that best describes how you really are, not how others see you or how you would like them to see you.

1. When solving a problem, I am precise and methodical.
2. When solving a problem, I like to consider all the possible alternatives.

3. When dealing with a problem, I tend to look for the most logical solution.
4. When solving a problem, I look to see how each solution will affect the people involved.

5. It helps to talk a problem out with a friend.
6. I'd rather solve my problems by myself.

7. I'm usually comfortable making decisions.
8. Nothing is written in stone; I prefer to keep my options open as long as possible.

9. If the system works the way it is, don't change it.
10. There's always a better way to do something, and I want to find it.

11. When I'm with a depressed person, I feel uncomfortable and don't know what to say.
12. When I'm with a depressed person, I try to find ways to cheer him or her up.

13. I tend to be expressive and outgoing.
14. I tend to be reserved and quiet.

15. I prefer to give my own projects definite deadlines.
16. I don't mind deadlines, but I think they should be flexible.

17. I like step-by-step instructions.
18. I like figuring things out for myself.

19. When one of my pets is sick, I will treat it as any other case.
20. When one of my pets is sick, I will do anything and everything to help it, even if it doesn't seem very reasonable.

21. I'm usually lonely or bored when by myself.
22. I savor and seek time by myself.

23. It really bothers me when I'm late for an appointment.
24. I try to be punctual but often run a few minutes late to appointments.

25. In the veterinary clinic, I prefer the routine cases to the exotic ones.
26. In the veterinary clinic, I get bored with the straightforward cases and savor the rare or exotic problem.

27. When people ask for my advice, I'll give them an unbiased and direct answer.
28. When people ask for my advice, I'll try to find a way to help them without hurting their feelings.

29. I enjoy mixing and mingling at parties.
30. I prefer one-on-one conversations at parties.

31. I like to get things done.
32. I do procrastinate from time to time.

33. I'm a sensible person.
34. I'm an imaginative and creative person.

35. When I know what's right, I don't like to spend a lot of time hearing someone else's ideas.
36. Even when I know I'm right, I'll still be patient and listen to another person's ideas.

37. I'm usually easy for people to read.
38. I'm usually difficult for people to read.

39. I make lists of things to do.
40. Rather than being held to a list, I'd prefer to tackle the project that's most interesting at the time.

41. I like to take the tried-and-true approach when solving a problem.
42. I like to blaze a new trail when looking at a problem.

43. Most issues have a clear right or wrong answer.
44. Most issues do not have one right or wrong answer—the truth is somewhere in between.

45. I like variety and action.
46. I prefer quiet and order.

47. When I've purchased something, I'm usually satisfied it was the right choice.
48. When I've purchased something, I often experience buyer's regret.

49. I take life as it is and don't spend a lot of time trying to change the world.
50. I often think about ways to make things better or change the world.

51. It's a greater compliment to be seen as tough, just, and fair.
52. It's a greater compliment to be seen as tender, merciful, and empathetic.

53. I'm usually pretty easy for people to get to know.
54. I'm usually pretty difficult for people to get to know.

55. I want to take charge of a situation and get it under control as soon as possible.
56. I'd rather observe the situation for a while before making any decisions.

57. I like to master or refine one skill before learning a new one.
58. I like to learn new skills, even if I haven't mastered the old ones yet.

continues

FIGURE 12.1   Personality Assessment, continued

59. I think it's fun to argue or debate issues.
60. I avoid arguments and debates.

61. I'm more of a talker than a listener.
62. I'm more of a listener than a talker.

63. I like life to be planned and structured.
64. I like life to be spontaneous and easygoing.

65. I'd rather work to solve a problem than spend all day thinking about solutions.
66. I like brainstorming solutions—the actual work of solving a problem is boring.

67. People usually see me as cool and reserved.
68. People usually think I'm kind-hearted.

69. I don't spend a lot of time worrying about things.
70. I'm a worrier.

71. I prefer to have a set schedule and stick to it.
72. I like walk-in appointments or emergencies; they keep the day interesting.

73. I like to work with people who don't rock the boat.
74. I don't mind when coworkers challenge the status quo to try to make things better.

75. I'm motivated by personal achievement.
76. I'm motivated by appreciation or recognition.

77. I have many close relationships.
78. I have a few close relationships.

79. I'd rather not start a new project until I've finished the old one.
80. I love starting new projects, even if they take time away from my current ones.

81. I need to see it to believe it.
82. I trust my intuition.

83. I don't tend to take criticism too personally.
84. I tend to take criticism very personally.

85. I like being noticed by others.
86. I prefer to work behind the scenes.

87. If I expect to wait for a while, I'll bring a book or something to do.
88. I don't worry about whether I'll be kept waiting—I'm sure I'll find something there to entertain me.

TABLE 12.1 Personality Assessment Score Sheet

Step 1: Circle the numbers that correspond to your answers.
Step 2: Add up the number of circles in each column, and write that number in the shaded row.
Step 3: Circle the two letters with the highest scores on each side of the center line.

1	2	3	4	5	6	7	8
9	10	11	12	13	14	15	16
17	18	19	20	21	22	23	24
25	26	27	28	29	30	31	32
33	34	35	36	37	38	39	40
41	42	43	44	45	46	47	48
49	50	51	52	53	54	55	56
57	58	59	60	61	62	63	64
65	66	67	68	69	70	71	72
73	74	75	76	77	78	79	80
81	82	83	84	85	86	87	88
A	B	C	D	E	F	G	H

TABLE 12.2   Personality Assessment Results

Cognitive Style	Social Style
A + C = Hawk	E + G = Leader
A + D = Dog	E + H = Energizer
B + D = Kitten	F + G = Engineer
B + C = Owl	F + H = Dreamer

Conclusion

As mentioned earlier, people are complicated creatures. One interesting thing about this assessment is that the same person can come up with different answers depending on the perspective from which he or she takes the test. If you answer the preceding questions from the perspective of "how I act at work," you may come up with a different social-cognitive style than if you answer from the perspective of "how I am at home."

This shouldn't come as a shock to you—most people aren't exactly the same person at work as they are at home. The variability in social-cognitive styles is further evidence of how complex we humans really are.

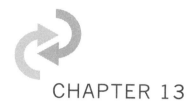

CHAPTER 13

Field Guide to Veterinary Personality Types

Social style is most important when dealing with someone on a day-to-day basis. So, it's pertinent when you're a veterinarian trying to understand how your own social style affects your daily interaction with the staff or your personal life. In this chapter, I provide a brief overview of how social styles tend to play out in the veterinary world and explore in more depth their relation to specific cognitive styles.

- *Leaders:* If you're a Leader, you tend to be an influencer and coach in the work setting. You're talkative and decisive. You want to take charge—and you expect people to follow!

- *Engineers:* As an Engineer, you're a reserved problem solver in the veterinary clinic. You gather information and make few suggestions, but when you speak people do listen, because you have great insight. You tend to focus on details or specific situations; you're not trying to change the entire clinic, just particular aspects of it.

- *Energizers:* If you're an Energizer, you often tinker with the status quo in the workplace, trying to make things better and get things done. You're action oriented and tend to spur others into action as well.
- *Dreamers:* If you're a Dreamer, you may seem like a quirky artist or wallflower, but you offer so much more. You have a strong value system and want the world to conform to your view. Dreamers don't fight every battle, but behind the scenes you may be quietly campaigning for change.

Combo Platter

Just as with cognitive styles, there are no absolutes in social style. People may have a personal preference among the four social styles, but they can adopt and adapt to another social style, based on the situation.

Most people aren't extreme in their type preferences and are in fact a blend of the outgoing Leader-Energizer or contemplative Engineer-Dreamer.

Veterinary Personality Types: What Your Social-Cognitive Styles Combination Says About You
Hawks: "Sense and Sensibility"

If you are a Hawkish veterinarian, you're an efficient, no-nonsense animal health care machine. You excel at using the resources available and working within the constraints placed on you by your clients. In fact, these limitations provide energizing challenges for the Hawkish veterinarian.

If you are a Hawkish veterinarian, you're an efficient, no-nonsense animal health care machine.

On the flip side, Hawks tend to have a do-it-yourself approach, so you may not always delegate well or train your staff to shoulder some of the burden. This self-sufficiency can create a bottleneck of care, because you're doing all of the work.

Hawks are logical decision makers who solve problems coolly and impassively. If you're a Hawk, you may be slow to adopt new treatments and medications, instead relying on the tried-and-true approach. Once a new product's benefits have been clearly explained, however, you're a converted and enthusiastic fan.

Hawks are decisive and work well in fast-paced settings, such as emergency clinics or busy veterinary practices. Hawks thrive on crisis and need lots of varying sensory input (data), so a spay clinic may not meet your career needs.

Work comes first—to a fault. Most Hawks don't see the value in play, so you may seldom engage in it. You can compulsively strive for efficiency, which may anger and annoy the staff. You can micromanage and push others too far, because not everyone shares the Hawk's value system.

Hawks don't deal well with emotional displays, so you may need to learn to express empathy to your clients. Hawks can seem cold when euthanizing a pet, especially when it is the right thing to do (because it doesn't naturally occur to them to express empathy when they are doing the right thing).

Leader Hawk

If you're a Leader Hawk, you're the classic take-no-prisoners boss. Leader Hawks are outgoing, and they get things done and get them done quickly. If you are a Leader Hawk, you can be forceful to get others to do what you want.

If staff members aren't ready to assume their role as a cog in the veterinary machine, then you may toss them out or criticize them in front of everyone else. This public flogging creates anxiety and low esteem among the staff. Staff may work hard to comply with the expected demands, but their level of commitment to the practice (or to you) may not meet your standards.

If you're a Leader Hawk, you're most comfortable with order and tradition and tend to make your decisions on this basis. "That's the way we've always done it" may be your mantra. This doesn't mean that you won't grow and learn professionally; you just need clear data that show the benefit of a particular drug or course of action.

Leader Hawks are most interested in general practice, internal medicine, or psychiatry. Leader Hawks make excellent businesspeople, and this is often the career path that they choose.[160–162]

Energizer Hawk

The exception to the Hawk's "work comes first" rule is when the Hawk is a strong Energizer. If you're an Energizer Hawk, you tend to be much more spontaneous than your Hawkish brethren and can almost be Kittenlike in your quest for fun. The most extreme Energizer Hawks can be risk takers and at times seem to live for the moment. Just the same, most Hawks aren't reckless and still tend to be very pragmatic about what they do in the clinic setting.

Energizer Hawks are great at making things happen and engaging staff in participating. If you're an Energizer Hawk, you make fast decisions based on the information in front of you. However, if you don't feel a sense of urgency to make a particular decision, you may not make it—for example, you probably won't repaint the exam room until the paint is peeling off the walls.

Energizer Hawks are the salespeople of the veterinary world. If you're an Energizer Hawk, you're great at selling your ideas to others and influencing people to do what you want, and you tend to create a loyal client base that has a cultlike devotion.

Energizer Hawks are sensory-based, outgoing, and always looking for new excitement, which is why they are thrill seekers. As an Energizer Hawk, you must feel a sense of urgency and be shown how your actions will have a positive, beneficial impact. Unlike most Hawks, Energizer Hawks don't usually think strategically. You may not look too far into the future; instead, you'll invest all of your efforts into the one case that challenges you. You need to learn to pace yourself.

It shouldn't come as a surprise that thrill-seeking Energizer Hawks handle the uncertainties of surgery and emergency medicine very well.[160–162]

Engineer Hawk

If you're an Engineer Hawk, you bring all of the good traits of this social-cognitive style to the table: decisiveness, systematic processes, and persistence. However, you're slow to change direction unless the evidence that you need to do so is clear and abundant. Acceptance of a new drug or different treatment approach will take a stack of published studies for you to absorb on your own.

As an Engineer Hawk, you're confident, loyal, and productive, with generally excellent record-keeping skills and thorough case workups. However, your only focus is the case—and this can mean that you keep staff after hours on a regular basis or come across as a dictator when you deliver instructions to your employees. You may also have difficulty praising staff, which is a problem in veterinary practice, where wages tend to be lower than in other health professions, and the esteem that staff derive from the work is an important part of their job satisfaction.

This personality type makes for excellent behind-the-scenes veterinarians, but Engineer Hawks' quiet competence doesn't always instill confidence in their clients. They need to be more outgoing and social to win the client over. These folks are often intrigued by specialties such as pathology and research.[160–162]

Dreamer Hawk

If you're a Dreamer Hawk, you're constantly observing and processing things, but seldom share your findings with others. You can seem reclusive or intensely private. However, once you've decided to weigh in on an issue, you'll quickly roll up your sleeves and show people how it should be done.

Most of the time, Dreamer Hawks are content to live in their own world. If people want a response from you, they'll have to explain why there's a need for immediate action. If there isn't a perceived need, you'll keep your head in the clouds. Dreamer Hawks may try to do it all themselves, which can affect the success of their business.

When a Dreamer Hawk has a mission or a goal, watch out! You tend to delegate most tasks only to others whom you perceive as competent, often ignoring or bulldozing the rest of the staff who is in your way. This lack of concern for the feelings of others in the work group can create friction after the job is done and the dust has settled.

Dreamer Hawks are drawn to anesthesiology, which makes sense because it balances the need for data and logic with the ability to be open-ended; new data are always coming in, depending on where the patient is in the surgery.[160-162]

Dogs: "Why Can't We All Just Get Along?"

The Dog is the ultimate feel-good movie personified. Dogs strive to create harmony, acceptance, and kindness around them. If you're a Dog, you have a loyal fan base of clients who can tell how much you care.

Because the interaction with pets and clients is reward in itself, you don't need a huge caseload or an intense clinic setting to be happy. In fact, you probably function better when there aren't demands to rush on to the next patient, so you can enjoy what you're doing then and there.

The Dog is born to please, and you'll try to respond to your clients' needs as much as possible. You determine a course of action based on the best choices for all involved—the pet and the owners. Dogs' desire to please can be a double-edged sword, because Dog veterinarians are those most likely to consistently discount their fees and give away their services.

> *Dogs' desire to please can be a double-edged sword . . . [they] are most likely to consistently discount their fees and give away their services.*

Because of their sensitive nature, Dogs are more likely to have emotional lows during their career. Invariably, a case doesn't go well or you'll have to deliver bad and unexpected news to a client, or there'll be an issue with a staff member. Whenever there is discord or strong negative emotions, you want to hide until the storm has blown over.

As a boss, you can be easily taken advantage of by less considerate or more self-serving staff members. Because Dogs naturally try to avoid conflict, problems will often get worse, especially when the rest of the staff is mad because the bad employee is being handled with kid gloves.

Leader Dogs

Leader Dogs create a warm, cohesive atmosphere. If you're a Leader Dog, you want everyone to get along and will work diligently to make your corner of the world (or work) its own little nirvana. Leader Dogs love having clinic get-togethers, which can become annoying to those who don't share this cognitive-social style combination.

Your style is supportive, and you truly care about everyone—sometimes forgetting to take care of yourself. Like most Dogs, you don't like conflict, which may frustrate the group if you don't manage problem employees directly.

As a Leader Dog, you may be needy in terms of wanting appreciation and recognition for what you've done. You're easily damaged by criticism and can be somewhat passive-aggressive; you mope around so much after being criticized that staff may find this worse than the behavior that prompted the critique. In human medicine, Leader Dogs are drawn to pediatrics; on the veterinary side, they'll likely excel in a slow- to medium-paced general practice.[161]

Energizer Dogs

If you're an Energizer Dog, you're socially outgoing, want to make a difference, and love entertaining the group. You may be the clown of the clinic, and you're usually making fun of yourself to keep everyone happy and motivated. To put your full energy behind a task or decision, you need to understand how it's relevant; otherwise, you'll just crack a few more jokes, and the ensuing laughter affirms your worth more immediately than working.

If the problem is social in nature, then you'll quickly try to address the issue, but won't do so head-on. In other words, if there is conflict in the clinic, you may try to lighten the mood rather than deal with the underlying problem.

The most fun-loving of all types, Energizer Dogs tend to live in the moment and don't worry about the consequences as much as they should. Although you can be the life of the party, your endless pursuit of fun can become tiresome at work.

If you're an Energizer Dog, you're so motivating and entertaining that you tend to keep multiple projects moving forward at one time by encouraging others to chip in and help. If you aren't getting the job done, then you need help to find the fun in your work.

In the clinic setting, an Energizer Dog makes a great emergency veterinarian. You love changes in the routine. You're also in tune with your team's strengths and weaknesses and manage to draw the best out of each team member. In the medical field, Energizer Dogs are often drawn to academia.[160–162]

Engineer Dogs

These quiet, relationship-oriented people are all about making choices that ensure safety and comfort without inconveniencing or harming anyone. If you're an Engineer Dog, "Dedication to Duty" is probably your motto. You can be a slow decision maker as you determine whether a particular course of action is beneficial to all. You're a tireless worker with a shy but cooperative disposition. Your social-cognitive style combination creates the ultimate team player. You're good at giving credit and recognition to others—sometimes to a fault, letting others take credit for your work.

If you're an Engineer Dog, you have very high standards and expectations of yourself and others. Unfortunately, if someone fails to live up to your standards, it will take a long while before you trust this person again. Engineer Dogs can also be troubled by ambiguity and may become frustrated by the challenging patient with problems that fall outside the typical caseload.

Because they're introverts, Engineer Dogs tend to bottle up their issues—creating a huge blowout when they finally do share what is bothering them. If you are an Engineer Dog, create an opportunity for a little pressure release along the way and avoid the festering abscess.

Anesthesiology dominates the Engineer Dog's career choices. The need for clear cause-and-effect consequences combined with empathy makes this an attractive specialty to Engineer Dogs.[160–162]

Dreamer Dogs

Dreamer Dogs go in as many different directions as a Labrador retriever puppy. If you're a Dreamer Dog, you're creative and artistic and can seem erratic as you bounce all over the place, reprioritizing as you go. You're so open-ended that you have a difficult time finishing a task. There's always something else more interesting or more important that you could be doing. You're very sensitive to your environment, which can make you seem unpredictable or unreliable because you keep changing what you're doing to make everyone happy.

If you're a Dreamer Dog, you're typically an easygoing person. You're naturally accepting of others, which may cause the more skeptical types to wonder what your ulterior motive is—but there isn't one.

Dreamer Dogs are probably the clinic therapists—someone people go to when they want to share a problem without worrying about judgment or criticism. You may not have many inherent leadership traits, but you still seem to blame yourself whenever something goes wrong at work. You do best in positions without high accountability.

Dreamer Dogs create an encouraging work environment. If you're surrounded by a good staff that is self-motivated, this arrangement can work. However, if your staff needs constant direction or supervision, you may quickly bog down and become unproductive, partly because you may not have managed the situation and partly because you may be stuck in a cycle of self-punishment.

Dreamer Dogs have an "if you build it, they will come" attitude toward creating a good workplace. Sometimes that works with employees; sometimes it doesn't. In most cases, you should have an office manager with a complementary personality type—and he or she needs to recognize the value in working with an opposite personality type (the Leader social style will complement the Dreamer social style nicely).

Dreamer Dogs are also those most easily manipulated by clients into discounting services so that they can afford to treat their pet. Rescuers fall into the Dreamer type, and there are always animals to rescue in a veterinary clinic. Dreamer Dogs are commonly found in either anesthesiology or general practice.[160–162]

Kittens: "I'm Okay, You're Okay"

Living in an abstract world, Kittens don't need hard data to make a decision, and they don't think linearly; instead, they use their innate sense of what's right and what's wrong to gather information and run it through an empathy filter to see how their decisions will affect others.

If you're a Kitten, you're accepting and nonjudgmental by nature and allow others to express themselves and do things their own way. You see the world as full of possibilities and celebrate creativity and individuality. The Kitten is the most idealistic and altruistic of the cognitive styles; Kittens are guided by a set of personal ethics and want to provide some sort of service to their community or humanity.

> *Kittens don't need hard data to make a decision . . . they use their innate sense of what's right and what's wrong to gather information.*

You tend to be excellent at interpreting the moods and body language of those around you. You're very aware of the social dynamics around you, which makes you an excellent persuader and motivator. Because Kittens' decision making isn't founded in sensory data or logic, you may have a difficult time explaining why you made the decision that you did.

Kittens are challenged by a lack of harmony and seek to avoid conflict. The culture of the workplace is important to you, because you'll be miserable if the work environment conflicts with your personal ideals.

Leader Kittens

As a Leader Kitten, you're in charge, outgoing, and socially adept. Leader Kittens are usually excellent at sales and convincing others that they need a product or service.

Leader Kittens have a high need to please but also an intuitive understanding of what it takes to improve a situation or solve a problem. Generally, you're upbeat at work and have an all-for-one-and-one-for-all approach. Most Kittens don't impose their value system on others, but those who are Leaders can become frustrated and angry if their advice isn't followed. Leader Kittens are an ironic group because they are easily upset if their value system is ignored, even if they were imposing their own values on others. As a Leader Kitten, you're an excellent teacher, mentor, or coach, and you can inspire others to achieve new heights. You're also very good at including everyone in social situations.[160–162]

In the clinic setting, you can function very well at almost any level. You get along well with others (so long as everyone is on the same page), and you have an eye toward keeping the workplace safe and fun. You're great at drawing the best out of those around you.

Leader Kittens, however, can be insecure and prone to emotional highs and lows if any workplace strife occurs. As a Leader Kitten, you may tend to personalize disagreements, creating unnecessary conflict and possibly making the situation worse. You may also work in bursts of energy, which can limit your productivity.

Leader Kittens aren't common among veterinarians, but in practice they can make excellent bosses, so long as they can set the tone.[173] Leader Kittens do not share their vision well, and if you're an associate in a practice whose owner is a different personality type, you may experience conflict.

Leader Kittens do a great job of being in tune with their clients, and their intuitive nature can make them excellent diagnosticians once they have the practical experience. Leader Kittens are predominantly drawn to teaching and academia.[161,162]

Energizer Kittens

The Energizer Kitten is the playful kitten zipping around the clinic. Gregarious and fun-loving, Energizer Kittens throw themselves full throttle into a task—so much so that they play hard until they crash and then need to recharge for a while.

If you're an Energizer Kitten, you have an enthusiasm that is contagious, and this enthusiasm often provides all of the necessary motivation to move a team to success. However, Energizer Kittens tend to leap before they look, which sometimes means your ideas are in for a rough landing. Ouch!

Energizer Kittens (who are energetic, intuitive, empathetic, and indecisive) can come across as unfocused or vacuous at times, as they jump from one topic or task to another. This misconception can create problems for you. You're also the type most likely to unwittingly send out flirty vibes, just because you're so good at reading people and saying what others want to hear.[160–162]

As an Energizer Kitten, you're inspirational, and you're among the best at brainstorming when a problem needs to be solved. However, you may not follow through with the solution—you'll be on to three or four other tasks before that problem is solved!

A lot of Energizer Kittens pursue a career in general practice.[160–162]

Engineer Kittens

Engineer Kittens are part kitten and part worker bee. If you're an Engineer Kitten, you're kind-hearted, dependable, and motivated to make things better. You're tireless in the pursuit of a goal but can face conflict when asked why you're doing things a certain way—especially by the Hawks and Dogs who rely more on sensory input (data) than on intuition.

Because you care so much, you can at times end up with a martyr complex—feeling that you're the only one who understands and can solve problems, but that you're unappreciated for this.[161] You also shy away from conflict or potential conflict, looking more like an ostrich than a Kitten.

Intellectually, you're seldom matched; Engineer Kittens' theoretical, intuitive nature allows them to excel in academia as researchers and teachers. Because you're a deep thinker, you can at times make the simplest thing too complex, losing the more concrete thinkers along the way. Engineer Kittens are very idealistic; this makes you an excellent champion of a cause that fits your value system, but it also leaves you prone to severe depression when your cause doesn't succeed. Like other Kittens, you tend to take criticism too personally.

In the workplace, you can be hard to know. With your introverted and intuitive preferences, you lead a rich inner life, and you don't usually share it with others.

In the exam room, Engineer Kittens approach cases as a counselor, guiding clients through the list of problems and solutions for their pet. However, you can come across as too theoretical and sometimes confuse the client. You tend to be very insightful when it comes to determining owners' motivations and willingness to pursue treatment for their pet. You read people well, which makes you effective at tailoring therapeutic plans that meet owners' needs, yet you're not so emotionally needy that you'll cut corners just because the client wants you to.

Engineer Kittens are most interested in internal medicine.[160–162]

Dreamer Kittens

The most idealistic of the 16 personality types, Dreamer Kittens need a cause to believe in—preferably one that will bring peace on earth and harmony to all. As such, they don't function well in a negative environment. They are natural-born healers.

If you're a Dreamer Kitten, you may have a tendency to overcommit. You may try to attend every school's career day, see your caseload, and be involved in a civic group, which can lead to exhaustion and depression because you just can't seem to keep up. Dreamer Kittens do not make strong administrators, so you'll need a good office manager to make sure your ship stays on course.

In the clinic, you only need to find value in your work to be properly motivated. However, you'll shut down if there's interpersonal conflict. You tend to keep things to yourself and hope for the best, but eventually Kitten rage will be seen if the problem signs aren't recognized and addressed.

As a coworker, you tend to be easygoing and unobtrusive. When you're in charge, however, you can be overly controlling if a subordinate's value system clashes with yours. You're a true believer in your cause, and you want others to follow suit. Although Dreamer Kittens can thrive in a variable environment (e.g., emergency clinic, behavior), you're also challenged to make quick decisions—you often want more information before choosing a direction.[160-162] You would find shelter medicine or working in canine physical rehabilitation to be good career options—each melds the need for a cause with enough variety to keep work interesting.

Owls

Learning without thought is labor lost; thought without learning is perilous.
—Confucius

No doubt about it, Confucius was an Owl. If you're an Owl, you're the most philosophical and conceptual of the cognitive styles. You absorb information from the world around you—seeing patterns and associations that others miss—and then develop a logical framework to understand and categorize those patterns.

As an Owl, you're a strategic thinker. You're self-confident and intellectual, trying to find and solve problems on a daily basis. Your goal is a deeper understanding of the world. However, you range from being a visionary to being an absent-minded professor—probably all on the same day. When you come across as a visionary, everyone follows your leadership. When you come across as an absent-minded professor, coworkers may drift in another direction. Because you're always looking beyond the horizon, you can seem either arrogant (solving problems that you think others can't) or scattered (worrying about things that haven't even happened yet).

Owls aren't sensitive or particularly empathetic, which may put you at odds with others in the clinic. Your innately logical decision making will seem cold and calculating to the Dogs and Kittens in the group. Left unchecked, you're likely to talk over clients' heads all day long. Why say "upset stomach" when you can more properly call it "gastroenteritis"? (Perhaps you should sit on your branch and ponder the meaning of effective communication—it isn't using big words.)

> *[Owls are] the most philosophical and conceptual of the cognitive styles.*

Leader Owls

The outgoing, visionary, problem-solving Owl is the prototypical leader. If you're a Leader Owl, you're a quick decision maker and are up to the debate when someone sees things differently than you do. You're happy to stick with and defend your position, but you're willing to change if a new pattern emerges during the debate. If you're a female Leader Owl, you can have issues resulting from gender bias even though you're competently in charge. This is because strong female leaders are often viewed as being arrogant, whereas the same traits in a male leader are simply interpreted as authoritative.

In the clinic setting, you may quickly rise to the level of supervisor or manager. You deploy employees as a general and motivate them to win the battle.[165] Because Leader Owls are so outgoing and direct, you can seem angry or confrontational to other personality types. This isn't your intent; you just don't feel the need to pussyfoot around an issue. You stand by your convictions and are willing to share them; if someone wants to change the way you think, then he or she must challenge you to a debate and win.

Although you're a strong leader, you also like to empower your coworkers to be independent-thinking problem solvers. You can become frustrated when dealing with people who don't want to think on their own, and this frustration may be perceived as impatience or insensitivity by staff. You need to remember that not everyone is an outgoing leader.

You may also broadcast your annoyance when you clearly see the solution to a problem but must wait for others to catch up. This reaction may give you an air of arrogance, and when accused of such behavior, you'll probably respond, "Well, I was right, wasn't I?"

As a Leader Owl, you can make a great practice owner or manager, but you may become very frustrated in a partnership or as an associate veterinarian. You want to set the pace and the vision, and you usually perceive others in a position of authority as either an annoyance or an inconvenience. You tend to expect excellence, not just competence, and may forget to provide the positive feedback that is important to keep staff members motivated.

Leader Owls are adept at thinking on their feet when things don't go well, so they function as well in emergency clinics as they do in other settings.[160-162] In a typical general practice, you might become bored unless you start asking deeper questions—looking for trends (what months does parvovirus peak and why?) and patterns (it rained a lot this winter; how will that affect pets with allergies?)

Energizer Owls

Energizer Owls are pioneers—using their abstract mind to explore the possibilities while looking for patterns in the universe. If you're an Energizer Owl, you'd rewrite the old adage to read "Invention is the mother of necessity." As an alternative thinker, you quickly infer the nature of a problem and set about trying to find possible solutions. You like to go through a brainstorming process—collecting all of the ideas, good and bad—before coming up with a final direction. You can slow down progress because you often play devil's advocate with new information to test its merit. (This contrary style, which is the thrill of intellectual pursuit to the Energizer Owl, simply annoys other types as being unnecessarily argumentative.)

In the clinic, you make an excellent veterinarian, but you may come across as competitive or challenging, so you need to learn to curb some of your enthusiastic inquiry when presented with someone else's ideas. You're decisive but retain an open-ended nature that allows you to choose another direction as more details emerge. Although Energizer Owls may be perceived as flaky, they're really attempting to do things in a better way. As an Energizer Owl, you'll have a reason for changing a policy or procedure and will have no problem educating others as to why they should adopt the new regimen. Because you're so problem-focused, you run the risk of alienating your coworkers. You need to learn to disagree without being disagreeable to maintain a productive workplace.

The Energizer Owl is commonly drawn to general practice.[160–162]

Engineer Owls

If you're an Engineer Owl, you're a strategizing mastermind—looking at the world as a four-dimensional chessboard and planning your attack far into the future.[165] An abstract but logical thinker, you're not concerned about the emotions of those around you. You're the most independent of the 16 types, not needing as much interaction with others as would a relationship-oriented Kitten or Dog. You can live in your own little logical world and be quite satisfied. Because Engineer Owls are so inwardly focused, you're more prone to conspiracy theories and suspicion. You take a cold, calculated look at a problem and find the most expedient and successful solution, regardless of the human cost. For example, Engineer Owls won't readily make allowances for the staff member who is having problems at home that are affecting his or her work performance. Their attitude will be "If he can't do the job, he shouldn't have the job."

In the clinic setting, you're very systematic. You'll develop checks and balances to make certain that cases are handled in a very specific way every time, and you'll look for ways to increase efficiency and effectiveness. You're a quick decision maker and can be extremely productive, but you also need coworkers who understand your personality; otherwise, they may think you're impersonal and overly analytical. You'll need an office manager with more empathetic tendencies and an open-door policy so that your staff has a friendly ear when needed.

Once you've settled on a path, you need considerable evidence to support a change in direction, because your original course was so thoroughly thought out. However, you're pragmatic to the core, and if the new direction can be proven to be more effective or efficient, then you'll be quickly converted.

As an Engineer Owl, you like creating solutions to life's big problems. You aren't as interested in the coworker who is always late or which cleaning agent is the best for the countertops, although you agree that these are important issues—for someone else to deal with.

Engineer Owls are perpetual students, which can be good in veterinary medicine, in which knowledge doubles every few years, but can be a problem if you're feeling stagnated or confined. If you aren't challenged, you'll choose another profession or find a more engaging clinic to work in. Not surprisingly, Engineer Owls are found in specialties such as neurology, research, pathology, and internal medicine.[160–162]

Dreamer Owls

Dreamer Owls are so busy dreaming up new ideas and ways of doing things that they often forget to share the brilliant solutions they thought of yesterday. If you're a Dreamer Owl, it can seem as though you're living in Never-Never Land, but you're actually trying to solve problems while you're there. You are independent and shy, which can make you seem rude, aloof, or forgetful. For example, Dreamer Owls are the people most likely to sneak out after the dinner party because they don't want to make a big scene when they say goodbye.

You're less comfortable in social situations, so you're usually drawn to science and architecture[162] rather than the healing arts, where you must interact with people constantly. You may shun office parties partly out of self-conscious shyness and partly because you have other things to do with your brain.

In the clinic setting, you can be full of great ideas if someone can get you to speak up. You're not very punctual and don't necessarily like to get a job done within a certain time frame—you'll probably spend half your time doing the job, and the other half trying to come up with a way to do the job better. One of the biggest problems with Dreamer Owls is that they spend too much time dreaming, neglecting to actually accomplish anything. This can make you a challenging coworker, because no one's ever sure what you're going to accomplish and when. Because you don't always function well with time constraints, you can make an excellent writer—your ability to see and articulate patterns gives you the gift of clarity and expression. You love the intellectual pursuit of the difficult case but will become bored with the routine. You're not a quick decision maker and can be challenged to come to a diagnosis in the process of a 20-minute appointment. You do best in specialty practice or a teaching hospital, where the most difficult cases are preselected for you and time constraints are less critical. Dreamer Owls also foster independent thinking in those around them—another good quality in a specialist or the faculty member. A lot of Dreamer Owls are interested in neurology, research, psychology, and pathology.[160–162]

How Veterinarians Compare with U.S. Norms by Personality Type

As a veterinarian, you already know that veterinarians march to a different drummer than much of the rest of society. A recently published study analyzed veterinary students (now presumably practicing veterinarians) over a 12-year period from 1996 to 2007 and compared their personality preference types with U.S. population norms.[173] Adapting the data to fit the personality categories discussed in this book provides insight into how the social-cognitive styles of the average veterinarian compare with those of the general U.S. population.

In terms of cognitive style, Hawks are the dominant species of veterinarian, making up nearly 40 percent of the profession. Moreover, veterinarians are usually Leader and Engineer Hawks—practical, no-nonsense, let's-make-a-decision-and-get-things-done types of people. The remaining 60 percent of veterinarians are divided fairly evenly across the other cognitive style types. What is most noteworthy is

Hawks are the dominant species of veterinarian, making up nearly 40 percent of the profession.

that the percentage of Owls among veterinarians is almost double that seen in the general U.S. population. The Owl cognitive style gives the profession a highly theoretical component.

Not altogether unsurprising, the profession has fewer Energizers and Dreamers than does the general U.S. population. Like it or not, veterinarians are not known for having a dynamic and outgoing nature like Energizers or for being artsy Dreamers. Instead, veterinarians seem to focus on fixing tangible problems and achieving measurable results. (See Table 13.1.)

Of course, all personality type preferences are represented in the profession—which is expected because (1) no two veterinarians are alike and (2) there's someone for everybody. Knowing about personality types may help you to understand why a client would rather see the other doctor in your practice. The other doctor likely communicates in a way that meets that client's needs. Bridging that gap, however, is the crux of this book: developing the means to recognize the client's communication needs rather than simply using your preferred conversation styles with every client.

The veterinary profession's largest area of disparity from U.S. population norms is with the Dog cognitive style—the data-driven, empathetic people. As discussed earlier, pet owners who are Dogs need a lot of reassurance that their relationship with their pet isn't going to be damaged by a course of action. With more than 40 percent of the U.S. population falling into the Dog category, yet only 23 percent of veterinarians indicating that type preference, the possibility of miscommunication is really likely unless veterinarians understand this group. Although it hasn't been studied, I would anticipate that Dogs also own the most pets because the Dog cognitive type is so much more relationship-oriented than the other cognitive types.

What has been documented is that empathetic and intuitive cognitive types (Dogs and Kittens) are more likely to oppose vivisection and animal research and more willing to make sacrifices for animals.[174] Some studies have suggested that

TABLE 13.1 Social-Cognitive Personality Types by U.S. Norm and DVM

Social Style	Cognitive Style (by percentage)				
	Hawk	Dog	Kitten	Owl	Total
Leader					
U.S. norm	8.7	12.3	2.5	1.8	25.3
DVM	12.8	7.0	4.2	4.9	28.9
Energizer					
U.S. norm	4.3	8.5	8.1	3.2	24.1
DVM	5.4	3.9	6.7	4.0	20.0
Engineer					
U.S. norm	11.6	13.8	1.5	2.1	29.0
DVM	12.8	7.7	4.9	4.6	30.0
Dreamer					
U.S. norm	5.4	8.8	4.5	3.3	22.0
DVM	3.4	4.5	4.8	5.5	18.2
Total					
U.S. norm	30.0	43.4	16.6	10.4	
DVM	34.4	23.1	20.6	19.0	

Adapted from Johnson, Gill, Grenier, and Taboada.[173]

Leader and Energizer Hawks are those who are least concerned about animal welfare, which is intriguing because these individuals make up 18 percent of the veterinary profession.[175]

Conclusion

Through the adaptation of data from a study of veterinary students over a 12-year period, you can now begin to get a sense of the social-cognitive types most drawn to the veterinary profession.[173] The average number of veterinarians who are Hawks and Owls is higher than that seen in the general U.S. population. But with Dogs and Kittens, the average number is lower. However, every personality type is represented in the profession.

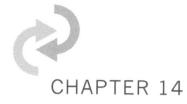

CHAPTER 14

Avoiding Conversation Quicksand

Now that you've learned to identify your clients' cognitive style and have gained some insight into your own personality type and conversation style, it's time to look at where you may get stuck in conversation quicksand with certain people. This is where it gets fun, because now you can start to modify and tailor your conversation style to meet your clients' needs, just as you develop a treatment plan to meet your patients' individual needs. I assume that you can communicate well with your own type and won't dwell on that.

Hawks Conversing with Other Types
Dogs

Danger signs flash whenever a Hawk doctor is talking to a Dog client. If Dr. Hawk doesn't move out of his or her comfort zone, the Dog client will regard him or her as cold and unfeeling.

Although Hawks and Dogs are both data-driven fact gatherers, they process that information in nearly opposite ways. A Dog needs a lot of reassurance and

How Hawks See Dogs

Hawks are likely to see Dogs in the following way:

- Emotional
- Illogical
- Irrational

To speak Dog, a Hawk needs to do the following:

- Talk about feelings
- Recognize how all are affected by the problem
- Apologize for bad news

empathy, and the Hawk is used to delivering just the facts. A Dog needs information to be packaged to emphasize the relationship with the pet—just talking clinically about an increasing blood urea nitrogen doesn't help a Dog understand the problem, but talking about how it makes the pet feel does make sense. It's important to follow up that knowledge with how the treatment plan will decrease the blood urea nitrogen so that the pet feels better again, too.

Hawks tend to treat clinical problems with a tried-and-true, systematic approach. When a cat is suspected of having diabetes, Hawks will do bloodwork and a urinalysis, change the cat's diet, start the cat on a dose of insulin, and perform follow-up lab work at a specific date. The Hawks do this because it's what they always do, and the approach achieves consistently good results. Unfortunately, a Dog doesn't want to hear "That's how I always do it." Dogs need a diagnostic and treatment plan that is seemingly tailored for their pet. Even if the plan isn't unique, savvy Hawks will make it appear as though they've designed the game plan with this specific owner in mind.

Kittens

The exact opposite of Hawks, Kittens will be turned off by Hawks' focus on test results or data and their very clinical approach to dealing with the problem. Hawks are likely to be annoyed that the Kitten keeps interrupting them and anticipating what they're going to say next. Kittens are associative thinkers; they don't process information sequentially like Hawks. Give them a broad outline and then help them color in the picture; don't focus on the details.

Kittens are also extremely sensitive to being judged, and it's important for Hawks to avoid language that makes it sound like the Kitten waited too long or didn't address a problem properly. Kittens' live-and-let-live lifestyle applies to their pets, too, and they don't want to impose on them.

Kittens may allow their dog to eat whatever it wants because the dog likes it. Explaining the cold hard facts of pancreatitis to Kittens isn't going to resonate with them. Instead, Hawk veterinarians need to talk about how the pet feels when it has pancreatitis and can't live life to its fullest. Explain how an alternative (not *better*—that sounds judgmental) diet will not make the pet feel sick; instead, it will enable the pet to run and play and be happy. Paint the big picture for Kittens, and they'll get your point.

> ## How Hawks See Kittens
>
> Hawks are likely to see Kittens in the following way:
>
> - Flaky
> - Unfocused
> - Unrealistic
>
> To speak Kitten, a Hawk needs to do the following:
>
> - Use analogies
> - Brainstorm solutions together
> - Paint a big picture

Owls

The Owl cognitive style will drive a Hawk crazy, because Owls want to focus on the bigger picture, at times ignoring their pet's immediate problem. Owls are likely to ask about every possible diagnostic test that could be run and want a breakdown as to the sensitivity and specificity of each test. This isn't because Owls are actually considering having the Hawk run all these tests on their pet—they're just curious.

Hawks are much more businesslike and will quickly grow frustrated with Owls' time-consuming and distracting quest for knowledge. The challenge is to give Owls enough information to cover the big picture without having to draw the entire landscape.

> ## How Hawks See Owls
>
> Hawks are likely to see Owls in the following way:
>
> - Too theoretical
> - Asking the wrong questions
> - Wanting too much information
>
> To speak Owl, a Hawk needs to do the following:
>
> - Give a broad overview
> - Discuss the diagnostic plan and process
> - Acknowledge that there are always other possibilities

Owls are theoretical thinkers, and Hawks tend to be much more practical. If a pet is vomiting and Dr. Hawk mentions five possible causes of nausea, then Dr. Hawk should be prepared to discuss all five causes. Generally, it's better to provide a broader overview (e.g., by saying, "nausea could be caused by [1] something he ate, [2] a metabolic problem inside, or [3] an infection"). If the cause of the nausea is something different from the three possibilities the Hawk mentioned, Owls aren't likely to think that the Hawk's made a mistake, because Owls are used to living in a world that has more options than most people realize.

Dogs Conversing with Other Types

Hawks

A Dog veterinarian is going to be too touchy-feely for the Hawk client, and friction is likely inevitable unless Dr. Dog changes his or her conversation style. Hawks will appreciate the information Dr. Dog shares but will roll their eyes at his or her focus on their pet's feelings.

How Dogs See Hawks

Dogs are likely to see Hawks in the following way:

- Cold, uncaring robots
- Overly concerned about costs
- Too demanding of action now

To speak Hawk, a Dog needs to do the following:

- Be organized
- Focus on outcomes of actions
- Directly address cost versus benefit of various plans

For example, when cancer has been diagnosed, the Dog veterinarian will talk about how the pet will feel during chemotherapy and afterward. The Hawk assumes that the pet will feel lousy during chemo and is much more interested in the logistics of treatment (how often and how much) and the success rates.

Dog veterinarians tend to present their information in stories about other animals and their personal experience. Hawks don't care. Give them research, give them data, give them Internet sites that have details.

The Dog's highly personal nature will directly conflict with the more impersonal and businesslike Hawk, and unfortunately, Hawks will often interpret the Dog's emotional (and heartfelt) information as being biased and, therefore, suspect.

Kittens

Kitten clients and Dog doctors generally get along well. A problem may arise when the Dog veterinarian advocates for a specific treatment plan that the Kitten doesn't want to put into play—and the harder the Dog pushes, the more likely the Kitten is to pull away.

Kittens and Dogs will be at odds on issues such as running lab work. Kittens don't live in a world of data—they can tell if their pet feels good or bad. So, running a follow-up urinalysis after treatment for a bladder infection isn't a priority for a Kitten, unless Dr. Dog can explain how serious an unresolved bladder infection can become (e.g., a blocked bladder, bladder stones, pyelonephritis).

> ## How Dogs See Kittens
>
> Dogs are likely to see Kittens in the following way:
>
> - Erratic
> - Disorganized
> - Out of touch with their pet's immediate needs
>
> To speak Kitten, a Dog needs to do the following:
>
> - Paint a picture of better health
> - Offer a variety of options
> - Not frame information in a way that will suggest the Kitten's actions or inactions are harming the pet

Dogs and Kittens both agree on the need for harmony in their world, and it's this common thread that needs to be communicated when reaching out to Kittens and trying to motivate them to take action. Dogs need to try to find and emphasize the fun for the pet. For example, "After we get a urine sample, I love to give dogs a special treat!"

Owls

In the case of Dogs and Owls, do opposites attract? Not likely. Although a Dog veterinarian is going to focus on how the pet is feeling now, the Owl client wants to know all about the future possibilities, theoretical causes and treatments, and pros and cons of any particular approach.

How Dogs See Owls

Dogs are likely to see Owls in the following way:

- Detached
- Too future-focused
- Wanting too much information

To speak Owl, a Dog needs to do the following:

- Provide a road map of the diagnostic or treatment plan
- Leave open the possibility that other options exist that haven't been considered
- Give Owls the resources to do their own homework, and invite them to discuss it further at a later date

To communicate best with Owls, Dogs need to present information in a framework that suggests they've considered all the possibilities. Just because it's allergy season and a pet is scratching doesn't mean it has allergies, at least according to the Owl.

So humor the Owl client. Use the dry-erase board and discuss the differentials for itchiness (no reason to use words like *pruritis* here just to impress the Owl); for example, list *skin infection, allergies,* and *dietary imbalance* on the board. Three or four possibilities ought to be enough.

Then, Dr. Dog should go through the findings of the physical exam and allow the Owl to see how he or she has systematically removed each possibility, leaving the obvious cause of the scratching as allergies. Now the Dog is ready to talk about treatment, and the Owl is convinced that Dr. Dog has done due diligence. It really isn't that hard to please Owls—just share the differential diagnosis list with them, and they'll be happy.

Kittens Conversing with Other Types

Hawks

The biggest challenge that a Kitten doctor and a Hawk client are going to face is discussing quality-of-life issues. A Hawk is likely to determine that the subcutaneous fluids, special diet, and Epogen injections aren't worth it if the cat's kidneys are going to fail anyway, and the Kitten doctor is going to be compelled to explain how the cat can have an excellent quality of life if those few steps are taken.

Even though Hawks do care about their pets, they look at life differently from Kittens and don't really understand their emotional perspective. In fact, the more

Dr. Kitten pushes for subcutaneous fluids and other palliative treatments, the more likely the Hawk will interpret this as a ploy to make money.

The reality is that 60 percent to 70 percent of Hawks are male, and if the Hawk is married, then the chances are good (60–70 percent) that his spouse is a Dog or Kitten.[161] Rather than pushing the Hawk on a treatment plan, send home the information about how treatment will enhance the cat's life, as well as an estimate of monthly costs. Your treatment plan will probably be accepted once that information has reached the spouse.

> ## How Kittens See Hawks
>
> Kittens are likely to see Hawks in the following way:
>
> - Impersonal
> - Worried only about money
> - Out of touch with their pet's needs and feelings
>
> To speak Hawk, a Kitten needs to do the following:
>
> - Focus on the known facts and the process for finding the unknowns
> - Explain how a treatment plan benefits the pet and costs less in the long run
> - Keep examples practical

Dogs

Dog clients will be frustrated when they ask the Kitten veterinarian how he or she arrived at a particular diagnosis and the reply is "It's the one that makes the most sense." Dogs are data-driven—they want to see, hear, feel, taste, and smell the problem. It may seem to the Dog as though Dr. Kitten pulled the diagnosis out of thin air, and even though Dr. Kitten is probably right, Dogs need some tangible data that they can process for themselves.

Kittens intuitively develop a list of differentials and then subconsciously cross each possibility off the list. For example, if the case involves a cat's litter box issues, Dr. Kitten's list is going to include urinary tract infection, bladder crystals or stones, and sterile cystitis. Dr. Kitten needs to show the Dog pet owner how a urinalysis will distinguish among the other differentials.

On an emotional level, the Dog client and the Kitten doctor are likely to get along well. Both want the pet to feel good and be happy. Both want the positive

How Kittens See Dogs

Kittens are likely to see Dogs in the following way:

- Wanting too many details
- Imposing their needs on the pet
- Challenging—everything has to be "proven" to them

To speak Dog, a Kitten needs to do the following:

- Explain how he or she arrived at a conclusion
- Give some specifics that the Dog can see for him- or herself
- Avoid threatening the relationship a Dog has with the pet

How Kittens See Owls

Kittens are likely to see Owls in the following way:

- Needing deeper explanations than necessary
- Too scientific and intellectual
- Less concerned about the pet and more about the process

To speak Owl, a Kitten needs to do the following:

- Provide a scientific framework to the discussion
- Present logical alternatives that can be supported with testing
- Send the Owl out the door with a list of good Internet sources for further study

relationship with the pet to be maintained. Kittens are more likely to be casual about answering some questions, which the Dog pet owner can perceive as not caring. For example, if the Dog asks which food is best and the Kitten answers, "There are a lot of great choices," the Dog will likely feel that's not a very thoughtful or specific answer. Instead, the Kitten needs to explain (in brief) how he or she determines the quality of a food and what the Dog should look for. As sensory-driven creatures, Dogs are going to love reading the ingredients label!

Owls

An Owl client is going to have a difficult time understanding a Kitten veterinarian. Even though they are both outside-the-box thinkers, Owls and Kittens process their information so differently that they can seldom find common ground. The Owl client wants patterns, trends, and theories; the Kitten doctor just wants to talk about this particular pet, how it is feeling, and what to do next.

A successful Kitten doctor will take a step back from focusing on the here and now and provide the Owl with an overview of the pet's problem. For a Kitten, the easiest way to do this is to discuss a few similar cases and how they were resolved. To be time-efficient, the Kitten obviously needs to condense some of the information presented to the Owl; after all, this isn't a symposium on pet health;

it's a 20-minute OFFICE call. If the Kitten has chosen the sample cases wisely, he or she will provide the Owl with what he or she needs to see the breadth of possibilities, and the Owl will trust that the Kitten sees the same landscape.

Owls Conversing with Other Types
Hawks

The only thing that keeps an Owl veterinarian from talking about theory and trends all day long is that he or she has another OFFICE call waiting in the adjacent exam room. This will lend some efficiency to the Owl's communication—and efficiency is the fuel that drives a Hawk.

Although they see the world differently, a Hawk will enjoy the Owl's logical approach to determining a diagnostic or treatment plan. In general, these two types communicate well in the exam room, so long as the Owl talks about the what and how instead of the why. Hawks just want to get down to brass tacks, and they trust that the Owl has considered all of the possibilities before he or she puts a plan into action. They don't want a play-by-play or a flowchart of how the Owl has reached a particular decision. If the end result adds up, then the Hawk is going to assume that the Owl has done the math right.

> ## How Owls See Hawks
>
> Owls are likely to see Hawks in the following way:
>
> - Pushing for results
> - Unwilling to explore the possibilities
> - Looking for simple explanations to complex problems
>
> To speak Hawk, an Owl needs to do the following:
>
> - Give specifics, not theories
> - Develop a game plan quickly
> - Talk about cause and effect

Dogs

Dogs can be troubled by Dr. Owl's far-sighted approach to their pet's problem. If the pet has a broken leg, the Dog client will want to know how the pet's going to feel during the healing process, what accommodations need to be made, and how this will affect the other people and pets in the household. Dr. Owl would prefer to simply

How Owls See Dogs

Owls are likely to see Dogs in the following way:

- Overly emotional
- Worried about the pet's feelings instead of the problem
- Unable to recognize that a particular course of action is going to lead to trouble (denial or wishful thinking on the Dog's part)

To speak Dog, an Owl needs to do the following:

- Acknowledge the owner's concern and worry
- Preface bad news with an apology (a warning) that he or she is about to deliver it
- Provide a treatment plan that emphasizes how it helps maintain the owner's relationship with the pet

discuss the healing time and how the dog will feel after the fracture has healed.

Owls have a tendency to deliver information with a detached, scholarly, almost robotic voice. It's as though they're narrating from the textbook and doing a bad job of it. This will really turn off Dogs, who want the Owl to see them and their pet for what they are: unique individuals, and not another of the 50 fractured femurs the Owl has treated in his or her career.

For success, Owls need to move out of their comfort zone and speak to their cognitive opposite with a feeling that doesn't come naturally. Owls aren't callous, but they tend to approach a pet's problem from such an academic perspective that they can seem detached. An Owl is likely to look at a badly fractured leg and smile, excited about the challenge of repairing it. Unfortunately, this great case is someone else's tragedy, and the owner is hurting as much emotionally as the pet is hurting physically. Owls need to take "empathy supplements" on a regular basis to communicate best with their Dog clients.

When Owls must deliver cold, hard facts, it's best if they open the discussion by apologizing for being blunt, but they need to share some unpleasant information with the owner. This helps Dogs shift gears (prepare for bad news) and keeps them from viewing the Owl as insensitive; after all, the Owl *was* sensitive enough to apologize.

Dog clients are not going to be interested in the trends and theories. Instead, they'll want concrete examples and are the first owners to ask, "What would you do if this was your pet?" An Owl communicating with a Dog should be prepared to answer this question with examples of similar cases to give the Dog an overview.

Kittens

Perhaps this book should've been called *Kittens Are from Venus, Owls Are from Mars.* That summarizes the dynamic between these two cognitive styles, which is to say there isn't much useful dialogue if they both insist on speaking their own language.

The Owl veterinarian and the Kitten client can communicate when they start to discuss possibilities. Kittens are all about experiencing life to its fullest and not stepping on anyone's toes in the process, so Owls need to talk about how a particular treatment plan will enhance the pet's quality of life.

Where these two cognitive styles will cross swords is if the Owl tells the Kitten that his or her actions are definitely going to cause a problem. Kittens live in the now and have a hard time thinking about future repercussions. However, Kittens can look back—so if a dog is getting fat, then it's possible to talk about how it's less able to walk as far now, partially because it's gained weight. Owls shouldn't be surprised or disappointed when the Kitten responds, "I can't walk as far, either." The Kitten is hearing the Owl, just in his or her own way.

Owls may be able to introduce the concept of trends (which appeals to them) by drawing an upward-sloping line in the air that shows the pet's weight over time. Without making any value judgments, Owls can simply point out that this weight will decrease the pet's overall strength and vitality. Owls can use sound bites to bring home their point, saying, for example, "Dogs who weigh less have been shown to live longer and be at a lower risk of diseases like cancer." Kittens hate sermons, so the Owl should make enough of a point to satisfy his or her Owlish needs, and then move on.

How Owls See Kittens

Owls are likely to see Kittens in the following way:

- Scattered and random
- Avoiding a frank discussion of the pet's issues
- Irrational

To speak Kitten, an Owl needs to do the following:

- Talk about the pet's quality of life with or without a treatment plan
- Enlist the Kitten's help by brainstorming solutions together
- Stay away from patterns, research, and theories

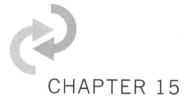

CHAPTER 15

Using Communication to Combat Burnout and Create Job Satisfaction

In short, he so buried himself in his books that he spent nights reading from twilight till daybreak and the days from dawn till dark; and so from little sleep and much reading, his brain dried up and he lost his wits.

—*Miguel de Cervantes,* Don Quixote

Burnout threatens everyone involved in the veterinary profession. When clinical practice is done right, with an intellectual and emotional investment by the practitioner, it's an extremely stressful profession.[176] Luckily, good communication skills can help diminish burnout to some degree.

Whereas stress is a normal physiologic response, burnout occurs when chronic stress leads to emotional, physical, or mental exhaustion. Burnout takes stress to a whole new level. Those suffering from burnout begin to feel overwhelmed and eventually have a difficult time keeping up with even the ordinary demands of daily life.

Unfortunately, burnout can affect any practitioner at any point in his or her career—in fact, young doctors are often more likely to become burned out than older ones.[177] The differences between stress and burnout are summarized in Table 15.1.[178] If you're concerned that you might be suffering from burnout, see the "Burnout Inventory" self-test in Appendix B.

TABLE 15.1 Stress Versus Burnout

	Stress	Burnout
Characterized by	Overengagement	Disengagement
Emotions are	Overactive	Blunted
Produces	Urgency and hyperactivity	Helplessness and hopelessness
Loss of	Energy	Motivation, ideals, hope
Causes	Anxiety	Detachment and depression
Primary damage	Physical	Emotional
End result	May kill you prematurely	May make life seem as though it isn't worth living

Adapted from Coping with Depression in the Ministry and Other Helping Professions *(Word, 1984). Used with permission.*

Factors that contribute to burnout include the following:[179,180]

- *Excessive workload:* Being pulled in too many directions to properly focus or feel effective
- *Lack of personal control:* Being in a workplace in which you have no decision-making ability; this is particularly challenging for the new practitioner, who may find the tests, treatments, medications, or management of his or her first practice to be deficient but is not empowered to improve the situation
- *Lack of recognition:* Feeling as though your efforts are not seen or appreciated; only hearing from the boss, clients, or staff when they have a criticism
- *Reduced career advancement opportunities:* Wanting to take on additional responsibilities but being stifled by the status quo, or feeling trapped in a certain

practice for various external reasons (e.g., spouse has a good job in the area; doesn't want to uproot kids from their school and move to a better practice in another town)

- *Poor leadership:* A boss who is a poor business manager, which creates a challenging situation for all who work in the practice (this burnout could affect the boss, too, who is a victim of his or her own poor leadership.)
- *Conflict:* feeling as though you have to fight a battle every day
- *Lack of balance in career and life:* Feeling as though there isn't enough time to do the job well and take care of yourself

One key antidote to burnout is career success.[181–183] The good news is that career success is something every veterinarian can create on his or her own, if he or she understands the key ingredients.[184,185] See the sidebar "The Six Ingredients of Career Success."

Read This Book

Many of the antidotes for burnout clearly have good communication as a common thread. In this book, I've shown how improved communication reduces conflict, improves compliance, and increases client retention and client satisfaction.[52] In other words, better communication increases job satisfaction, which then leads to even better communication and even greater satisfaction.[49]

Looking at the six elements of job satisfaction, it all makes sense: Work hard and do a good job, keep clients happy, make enough money to be comfortable, take enough time off to enjoy your friends and family, pursue personal goals, and remember that you aren't an island but a member of a caring profession; meet up with your colleagues and compare stories while working toward the greater good. In helping yourself, you'll help others.

Clients will always want you to be more available, work longer hours, take less time off, answer their phone calls, and so on. They don't mean to be selfish or demanding; they just respect the important role you play in their life and the lives of their pets.

The Six Ingredients of Career Success

As published in the *Journal of the American Veterinary Medical Association*, these are the six ingredients of career success:[50]

1. **Fulfillment from Work**
   - Developing nurturing professional relationships
   - Being honest about how much you and your staff can really accomplish in one day

2. **Balancing Relationships**
   - Developing clear boundaries between work life and personal life
   - Fostering personal relationships and keeping in touch with friends, family, and colleagues
   - Taking time off to recharge your battery—it's your responsibility to yourself, your family, and your patients

3. **Pursuing Personal Goals**
   - Taking breaks during the day, which can be as simple as going out for lunch or scheduling 20 minutes to play fetch with a boarding animal
   - Eating properly, exercising, and sleeping enough, which may seem an odd personal goal, yet it is not a reality for a lot of veterinarians
   - Getting up a few minutes earlier in the morning and reading a book or enjoying a quiet cup of coffee
   - Finding a hobby, and scheduling time for it
   - Having fun on a regular basis
   - Finding a relaxation technique that works for you
   - Realizing you have only two options: You can either change the situation, or you can change how you feel about it.

4. **Helping Others**
   - Studies have shown that those who take time away from work to help others and provide a service to humanity have higher levels of job satisfaction.[186–188]

5. **Making Enough Money**
   - Charge a fair fee for your services and stop giving them away.

- Let someone else on the staff deal with the money issues when talking with clients, so that you don't have to.
- Realize when you are making enough money and be content. In a 2008 survey of health professionals, 46 percent of the respondents stated that better communication and interpersonal relationships improved job satisfaction, whereas only three percent felt that more money (bonuses) alone would increase job satisfaction.[188]

6. **Participating in the Profession**

- Talk with colleagues at conferences and seminars; share war stories. Several studies have shown that practitioners who isolate themselves from colleagues are more likely to experience compassion fatigue and burnout.[161,189]
- Make colleagues part of your support system. After all, no one understands the stresses you are dealing with on a daily basis better than a fellow veterinarian. "One of the most effective ways of managing stresses associated with clinical practice is by participating in a supportive peer supervision group process."[190]

However, you've got to find the balance and stop to smell the roses every now and then. Although clients may be asking for more of your time, they're also assuming that you're taking the time you need to recharge your own batteries. This is your responsibility—to your own well-being, to your family, and to the animals you treat.

I hope this book will help you find more joy in day-to-day veterinary practice through better communication with clients and staff. However, achieving career success will likely mean balancing your life in nonveterinary ways—stepping out of the clinic every once in a while to gain a fresh perspective.

Yes, we should all aspire to be the best doctors possible, but I dare you to become known for more than just your skills as a healer: Give time and energy to your family and your community or risk having a tombstone that simply reads, "Here lies a good veterinarian."

Appendix A

Personality Assessment

Personality Assessment

Are you a Leader Dog, a Dreamer Kitten, or somewhere in between?

In each group of two questions, circle the number that best describes how you really are, not how others see you or how you would like them to see you.

1. When solving a problem, I am precise and methodical.
2. When solving a problem, I like to consider all the possible alternatives.

3. When dealing with a problem, I tend to look for the most logical solution.
4. When solving a problem, I look to see how each solution will affect the people involved.

5. It helps to talk a problem out with a friend.
6. I'd rather solve my problems by myself.

7. I'm usually comfortable making decisions.
8. Nothing is written in stone; I prefer to keep my options open as long as possible.

9. If the system works the way it is, don't change it.
10. There's always a better way to do something, and I want to find it.

11. When I'm with a depressed person, I feel uncomfortable and don't know what to say.
12. When I'm with a depressed person, I try to find ways to cheer him or her up.

continues

13. I tend to be expressive and outgoing.
14. I tend to be reserved and quiet.

15. I prefer to give my own projects definite deadlines.
16. I don't mind deadlines, but I think they should be flexible.

17. I like step-by-step instructions.
18. I like figuring things out for myself.

19. When one of my pets is sick, I will treat it as any other case.
20. When one of my pets is sick, I will do anything and everything to help it, even if it doesn't seem very reasonable.

21. I'm usually lonely or bored when by myself.
22. I savor and seek time by myself.

23. It really bothers me when I'm late for an appointment.
24. I try to be punctual but often run a few minutes late to appointments.

25. In the veterinary clinic, I prefer the routine cases to the exotic ones.
26. In the veterinary clinic, I get bored with the straightforward cases and savor the rare or exotic problem.

27. When people ask for my advice, I'll give them an unbiased and direct answer.
28. When people ask for my advice, I'll try to find a way to help them without hurting their feelings.

29. I enjoy mixing and mingling at parties.
30. I prefer one-on-one conversations at parties.

31. I like to get things done.
32. I do procrastinate from time to time.

33. I'm a sensible person.
34. I'm an imaginative and creative person.

35. When I know what's right, I don't like to spend a lot of time hearing someone else's ideas.
36. Even when I know I'm right, I'll still be patient and listen to another person's ideas.

37. I'm usually easy for people to read.
38. I'm usually difficult for people to read.

39. I make lists of things to do.
40. Rather than being held to a list, I'd prefer to tackle the project that's most interesting at the time.

41. I like to take the tried-and-true approach when solving a problem.
42. I like to blaze a new trail when looking at a problem.

43. Most issues have a clear right or wrong answer.
44. Most issues do not have one right or wrong answer—the truth is somewhere in between.

45. I like variety and action.
46. I prefer quiet and order.

47. When I've purchased something, I'm usually satisfied it was the right choice.
48. When I've purchased something, I often experience buyer's regret.

49. I take life as it is and don't spend a lot of time trying to change the world.
50. I often think about ways to make things better or change the world.

51. It's a greater compliment to be seen as tough, just, and fair.
52. It's a greater compliment to be seen as tender, merciful, and empathetic.

53. I'm usually pretty easy for people to get to know.
54. I'm usually pretty difficult for people to get to know.

55. I want to take charge of a situation and get it under control as soon as possible.
56. I'd rather observe the situation for a while before making any decisions.

57. I like to master or refine one skill before learning a new one.
58. I like to learn new skills, even if I haven't mastered the old ones yet.

59. I think it's fun to argue or debate issues.
60. I avoid arguments and debates.

61. I'm more of a talker than a listener.
62. I'm more of a listener than a talker.

63. I like life to be planned and structured.
64. I like life to be spontaneous and easygoing.

65. I'd rather work to solve a problem than spend all day thinking about solutions.
66. I like brainstorming solutions—the actual work of solving a problem is boring.

67. People usually see me as cool and reserved.
68. People usually think I'm kind-hearted.

69. I don't spend a lot of time worrying about things.
70. I'm a worrier.

71. I prefer to have a set schedule and stick to it.
72. I like walk-in appointments or emergencies; they keep the day interesting.

73. I like to work with people who don't rock the boat.
74. I don't mind when coworkers challenge the status quo to try to make things better.

75. I'm motivated by personal achievement.
76. I'm motivated by appreciation or recognition.

continues

77. I have many close relationships.
78. I have a few close relationships.

79. I'd rather not start a new project until I've finished the old one.
80. I love starting new projects, even if they take time away from my current ones.

81. I need to see it to believe it.
82. I trust my intuition.

83. I don't tend to take criticism too personally.
84. I tend to take criticism very personally.

85. I like being noticed by others.
86. I prefer to work behind the scenes.

87. If I expect to wait for a while, I'll bring a book or something to do.
88. I don't worry about whether I'll be kept waiting—I'm sure I'll find something there to entertain me.

Refer to Chapter 12 for more information, and see Tables 12.1 and 12.2 for scoring procedures.

Appendix B

Burnout Inventory

Burnout Inventory

If you believe you are headed for burnout, here is a way to test yourself for the symptoms of a downward spiral. Check those statements with which you agree.

☐ More and more, I find that I can hardly wait for quitting time to come so that I can leave work.

☐ I feel like I'm not doing any good at work these days.

☐ I'm more irritable than I used to be.

☐ I'm thinking more about changing jobs.

☐ Lately, I've become more cynical and negative.

☐ I have more headaches (or backaches, or other physical symptoms) than usual.

☐ I often feel hopeless, like "Who cares?"

☐ I drink more now or take tranquilizers just to cope with everyday stress.

☐ My energy level is not what it used to be. I'm tired all the time.

☐ I feel a lot of pressure and responsibility at work these days.

☐ My memory is not as good as it used to be.

☐ I don't seem to concentrate or pay attention as I did in the past.

continues

Burnout Inventory, continued

- ☐ I don't sleep as well.
- ☐ My appetite is decreased these days (or, I can't seem to stop eating).
- ☐ I feel unfulfilled and disillusioned.
- ☐ I'm not as enthusiastic about work as I was a year or two ago.
- ☐ I feel like a failure at work. All the work I've done hasn't been worth it.
- ☐ I can't seem to make decisions as easily as I once did.
- ☐ I find I'm doing fewer things at work that I like or that I do well.
- ☐ I often ask myself, "Why bother? It doesn't really matter anyhow."
- ☐ I don't feel adequately rewarded or noticed for all the work I've done.
- ☐ I feel hopeless, and I can't see any way out of my problems.
- ☐ People have told me I'm too idealistic about my job.
- ☐ I think my career has just about come to a dead end.

Count up your checkmarks. If you agree with most of these statements, then you may be feeling burnout and be in need of professional help or counseling or, at least, a change in lifestyle.

Adapted from Archibald Hart, Coping with Depression in the Ministry and Other Helping Professions *(Word, 1984). Used with permission.*

Appendix C

Hobby Suggestions Based on Social-Cognitive Styles

Hobby Suggestions Based on Social-Cognitive Styles

	Leader	Engineer	Energizer	Dreamer
Owl	Coach sports, service clubs	Become the leader of a club or organization for children (Boys and Girls Club, 4-H, Girl or Boy Scouts, etc.)	Become involved in a book club, service organization, politics	Take up a hands-on hobby—crafts, painting, or even skydiving
Kitten	Garden, cook	Visit museums, collect historical items	Take up theater or other performance art, service clubs	Compose, write a book, learn an instrument
Dog	Teach others, mentor, radio or television	Counsel others, correspond with friends, write poetry	Enjoy travel, politics, being champion of a cause	Enjoy being part of a group that makes things better, reading, music
Hawk	Lead civic groups, do fundraising	Repair clocks, paint, hands-on pursuits	Invent things, start household projects	Architecture, model building, sculpture

Adapted from Keirsey[165]

References

1. Milani, M. 2003. Practitioner-client communication: When goals conflict. *Canadian Veterinary Journal* 44(8): 675–78.

2. Timmins, R. P. 2006. How does emotional intelligence fit into the paradigm of veterinary medical education? *Journal of Veterinary Medical Education 33*(1): 71–75.

3. Hare, D. 2003. Good communication skills key to success. *Canadian Veterinary Journal* 44(8): 621–22.

4. Thompson, G., and J. Jenkins. 2004. *Verbal judo: The gentle art of persuasion.* New York: Quill.

5. Gayzer, K. 2009. Good communication isn't always what you think. *Clinicians Brief* 7(7): 25–27.

6. McGee, A. R. N. 20011. *Detailed discussion of veterinarian client issues.* East Lansing: Michigan State University College of Law.

7. Magrath, C., and G. Little, 2009. *Communication—A skill that needs to be acquired.* http://vetrecordjobs.com/vetrecordjobs/static/communication-a-skill-that-needs-to-be-acquired.html.

8. http://veterinaryconsumer.blogspot.com/p/veterinary-complaints.html.

9. Eastaugh, S. R. (2004). Reducing litigation costs through better patient communication. *Physician Executive Journal* 30(3): 36–38.

10. Shaw, J. R., B. N. Bonnett, C. L. Adams, and D. L. Roter. 2006. Veterinarian-client-patient communication patterns used during clinical appointments in companion animal practice. *Journal of the American Veterinary Medical Association* 228(5): 714–21.

11. Spickard, R. Is it always someone's fault? *News and Views*, September 2006.

12. Anderson, G. F., P. S. Hussey, B. K. Frogner, and H. R. Waters, 2005. Health spending in the United States and the rest of the industrialized world. *Health Affairs* 24(4): 903–14.

13. Brown, J. P., and J. D. Silverman. 1999. Current and future market for veterinarians and veterinary medical services in the United States: Executive summary. *Journal of the American Veterinary Medical Association* 215(2): 161–83.

14. Martin, E. A. 2006. Managing client communication for effective practice: What skills should veterinary graduates have acquired for success? *Journal of Veterinary Medical Education 33*(1): 45–9.

15. Levinson, W., R. Gorawara-Bhat, R. Dueck, B. Egener, A. Kao, C. Kerr, B. Lo, et al. 1999. Resolving disagreements in the patient-physician relationship: Tools for improving communication in managed care. *JAMA* 282(15): 1477–83.

16. American Pet Products Association. *Industry statistics and trends.* http://www.americanpetproducts.org/press_industrytrends.asp.

17.   Volk J. O., K. E. Felsted, R. F. Cummings, J. W. Slocum, W. L. Cron, K. G. Ryan, and M. C. Moosbrugger. 2005. Executive summary of the AVMA-Pfizer business practices study. *Journal of the American Veterinary Medical Association* 226(2): 212–18.

18.   Fouts, R. 2007. *Customer retention versus customer loyalty.* http://www.helium.com/items/491965-customer-retention-versus-customer-loyalty.

19.   http://www.80-20presentationrule.com/whatisrule.html.

20.   http://en.wikipedia.org/wiki/Pareto_principle#cite_note-2.

21.   Gordon, G. H., L. Baker, and W. Levinson. 1995. Physician-patient communication in managed care. *Western Journal of Medicine* 163(6): 527–31.

22.   Smith, C. 2009. Client satisfaction pays: Quality service for practice success. 2nd ed. Lakewood, CO: AAHA Press.

23.   Doctors' interpersonal skills are valued more than training. 2004. *Wall Street Journal Online,* September 28. http://online.wsj.com/article/SB109630288893728881.

24.   McCullough, S. 2003. Vetting a vet. *Washington Post,* December 7.

25.   Coe, J. B., C. L. Adams, and B. N. Bonnett. 2007. A focus group study of veterinarians' and pet owners' perceptions of the monetary aspects of veterinary care. *Journal of the American Veterinary Medical Association* 231(10): 1510–18.

26.   American Veterinary Medical Association. 2007. *2007 US pet ownership & demographics sourcebook.* Schaumburg, IL: Author.

27.   Wise, J. K., and A. J. Shepherd, 2003. Selection of a veterinarian by US pet-owning households. *Journal of the American Veterinary Medical Association* 223(8): 1121–22.

28.   Managing smart: Marketing mania. 2009. *Veterinary Economics* 50(8): 34.

29.   MacMillan, D. 2009. Does social media sway online shopping? http://www.businessweek.com/the_thread/blogspotting/archives/2009/08/does_social_med.html.

30.   BabyCenter Study Report. 2009. http://wwwbabycentersolutions.com.

31.   Facebook promotion does a small business good. *Veterinary Economics.* http://veterinarybusiness.dvm360.com/vetec/ArticleStandard/Article/detail/659625.

32.   Taylor, V. *A brand's Facebook fans are valuable consumers.* http://blogs.forbes.com/marketshare/2010/06/11/a-brand's-facebook-fans-are-valuable-consumers/.

33.   Ward, E. 2010. Social revolution: How Facebook, Twitter, and YouTube can help your veterinary practice. *Veterinary Economics* 51(2).

34.   Clark, K. 2010. Getting clients to comply. *Veterinary Record* 166(26): 805–7.

35.   Abood, S. K. Effectively communicating with your clients. *Topics in Companion Animal Medicine* 23(3): 143–47.

36.   Grave, K., and H. Tanem. 1999. Compliance with short-term oral antibacterial drug treatment in dogs. *Journal of Small Animal Practice* 40(4): 158–62.

37.   Barter, L. S., J. E. Maddison, and A. D. Watson. 1996. Comparison of methods to assess dog owners' therapeutic compliance. *Australian Veterinary Journal* 74(6): 443–46.

38.   Enhancing patient adherence: Proceedings of the Pinnacle Roundtable Discussion. 2004. *Highlights Newsletter* 7(4).

39. American Animal Hospital Association. 2003. *The path to high-quality care: Practical tips for improving compliance.* Lakewood, CO: AAHA Press.

40. *2009 AAHA Compliance Follow-Up Study.* Lakewood, CO: AAHA Press.

41. Communicate with clients to boost testing compliance. 2010. *Veterinary Economics* 51(2).

42. Jackson, J., and L. Bosse-Smith. 2008. *Leveraging your communication style.* Nashville, TN: Abingdon Press.

43. Klingborg, D., and J. Klingborg. 2007. Talking with clients about money. *Veterinary Clinics of North America* 37(1): 79–93.

44. Hickson, G. B., E. W. Clayton, P. B. Githens, and F. A. Sloan. 1992. Factors that prompted families to file medical malpractice claims following perinatal injuries. *JAMA* 267: 1359–63.

45. Holloway, J. D. 2003. Talking dollars. *Money Matters* 6(1): 1–2.

46. Milani, M. M. 1995. *The art of veterinary practice: A guide to client communication.* Philadelphia: University of Pennsylvania Press.

47. Holloway, J. D. 2003. Talking dollars. *Money Matters* 6(1): 1–2.

48. Borglum, K. 2004. Talking with patients about costs. *Sonoma Medicine* 55(2): 1–5. http://www.scma.org/magazine.scp/sp04/borglum.html.

49. Desmond, J., and L. Copeland. 2000. *Communicating with today's patient.* San Francisco: Jossey-Bass.

50. Ruby, K., and R. DeBowes. 2007. The veterinary health care team. *Veterinary Clinics of North America* 37(1): 19–35.

51. Lewis, R. E., and J. S. Klausner. 2003. Nontechnical competencies underlying career success as a veterinarian. *Journal of the American Veterinary Medical Association* 222(12): 1690–96.

52. Roter, D., and J. Hall. 2006. *Doctors talking with patients/patients talking with doctors.* 2nd ed. Westport, CT: Praeger.

53. Meadows, R. 2009. The human–animal bond: Client versus patient needs. *Clinician's Brief* 7(9).

54. Fox, J. 2010. *Responsibility, respect and relationships are important for patients.* http://www.kevinmd.com/blog/2010/12/responsibility-respect-relationships-important-patients.html.

55. Katz, J. 2003. *The new work of dogs: Tending to life, love, and family.* New York: Villard.

56. Ang, M. 2002. Advanced communication skills: Conflict management and persuasion. *Academic Medicine* 77(11): 1166.

57. Clack, G. B., J. Allen, D. Cooper, and J. O. Head. 2004. Personality differences between doctors and their patients: Implications for the teaching of communication skills. *Medical Education* 38(2): 177–86.

58. Clayman, M. L., A. U. Pandit, A. R. Bergeron, K. A. Cameron, E. Ross, and M. S Wolf. 2010. Ask, understand, remember: A brief measure of patient communication self-efficacy within clinical encounters. *Journal of Health Communication* 15(Suppl. 2): 72–79.

59. Ashbury, F. D., D. C. Iverson, and B. Kralj. 2001. Physician communication skills: Results of a survey of general/family practitioners in Newfoundland. *Medical Education Online* 6:1. http://www.med-ed-online.org/res00014.html.

60.   *Secret language divides doctors and patients.* 2002. http://www.peoplespharmacy.com/2002/04/15/secret-language/.

61.   Sevinc, A., S. Buyukberber, and C. Camci. 2005. Medical jargon: Obstacle to effective communication between physicians and patients. *Medical Principles and Practice* 14(4): 292.

62.   Sokol, D. K. 2008. Medicine as performance: What can magicians teach doctors? *Journal of the Royal Society of Medicine* 101(9): 443–46.

63.   Rehman, S. U., P. J. Nietert, D. W. Cope, and A. O. Kilpatrick. 2005. What to wear today? Effect of doctor's attire on the trust and confidence of patients. *American Journal of Medicine* 118(11): 1279–86.

64.   Royal Free Hospital Survey. *Postgraduate Medical Journal.*

65.   Newport, F. 1999. Landing a man on the moon: The public's view. Gallup News Service, July 20.

66.   Jones, V. A. 1999. The white coat: Why not follow suit? *JAMA* 281(5): 478.

67.   Gallagher J, F. Waldron Lynch, J. Stack, and J. Barragry. 2008. Dress and address: Patient preferences regarding doctor's style of dress and patient interaction. *Irish Medical Journal* 101(7): 211–13.

68.   Brandt, L. J. 2003. On the value of an old dress code in the new millennium. *Archives of Internal Medicine* 163(11): 1277–81.

69.   Sanders, T. 2005. *The likeability factor: How to boost your L-factor and achieve your life's dreams.* New York: Three Rivers Press.

70.   Holloway, P. *The secret to likeability.* http://www.aboutpeople.com/Articles/Likeability.php.

71.   Hall, J. A., T. G. Horgan, T. S. Stein, and D. L. Roter. 2002. Liking in the physician-patient relationship. *Patient Education and Counseling* 48(1): 69–77.

72.   Cousin, G., and M. Schmid Mast. 2011. Agreeable patient meets affiliative physician: How physician behavior affects patient outcomes depends on patient personality. *Patient Education and Counseling.* Epub ahead of print.

73.   Jayanti, R., and T. Whipple. 2008. Like me . . . like me not: The role of physician likability on service evaluations. *Journal of Marketing Theory and Practice* 16(1): 79–86.

74.   Beatles. The End. In *Abbey Road.* ©1969 Apple Records.

75.   Strand, E. B. 2006. Enhanced communication by developing a non-anxious presence: A key attribute for the successful veterinarian. *Journal of Veterinary Medical Education* 33(1): 65–70.

76.   Lenski, T. *Cultivating a non-anxious presence during difficult conversations.* http://lenski.com/conflictzen/non-anxious-presence-in-difficult-conversations/.

77.   Epstein, R. M. 2003. Mindful practice in action. I: Technical competence, evidence-based medicine, and relationship-centered care. *Families, Systems, & Health* 21(1): 1–9.

78.   Shaw, J. R., C. L. Adams, B. N. Bonnett, S. Larson, and D. L. Roter. 2008. Veterinarian-client-patient communication during wellness appointments versus appointments related to a health problem in companion animal practice. *Journal of the American Veterinary Medical Association* 233(10): 1576–86.

79.   Shaw, J. R., C. L. Adams, B. N. Bonnett, S. Larson, and D. L. Roter. 2004. Use of the Roter interaction analysis system to analyze veterinarian-client-patient communication in companion animal practice. *Journal of the American Veterinary Medical Association* 225(2): 222–29.

80. Dysart, L. M. A., J. B. Coe, and C. L. Adams. 2011. Analysis of solicitation of client concerns in companion animal practice. *Journal of the American Veterinary Medical Association* 238: 1609–15.

81. Gorawara-Bhat, R., and M. A. Cook. 2011. Eye contact in patient-centered communication. *Patient Education and Counseling.* Epub ahead of print.

82. Lill, M. M., and T. J. Wilkinson. 2005. Judging a book by its cover: Descriptive survey of patients' preferences for doctors' appearance and mode of address. *British Medical Journal* 331(7531): 1524–27.

83. Ambady, N., and R. Rosenthal. 1997. Judging social behavior using "thin slices." *Chance* 10: 12–18.

84. Ozono, H., M. Watabe, S. Yoshikawa, S. Nakashima, N. O. Rule, N. Ambady, and R. B. Adams. 2010. What's in a smile? Cultural differences in the effects of smiling on judgments of trustworthiness. *Letters on Evolutionary Behavioral Science* 1(1): 15–18.

85. Ambady, N., and R. Rosenthal. 1993. Half a minute: Predicting teacher evaluations from thin slices of behavior and physical attractiveness. *Journal of Personality and Social Psychology* 64(3): 431–41.

86. Jancin, B. 2001. Patients kept waiting want a simple apology. *Internal Medicine News.*

87. Frankel, R., and T. Stein. 1999. Getting the most out of the clinical encounter: The four habits model. *Permanente Journal* 3(3): 79–88.

88. de Haes, H., and J. Bensing. 2009. Endpoints in medical communication research, proposing a framework of functions and outcomes. *Patient Education and Counseling* 74(3): 287–94.

89. Cameron, K. A., H. de Haes, and A. Visser. 2009. Theories in health communication research. *Patient Education and Counseling* 74(3): 279–81.

90. Levinson, W., D. L. Roter, J. P. Mullooly, V. T. Dull, and R. M. Frankel. 1997. Physician-patient communication: The relationship with malpractice claims among primary care physicians and surgeons. *JAMA* 277: 553–59.

91. Beckman, H. B., K. M. Markakis, A. L. Suchman, and R. M. Frankel. 1994. The doctor-patient relationship and malpractice: Lessons from plaintiff depositions. *Archives of Internal Medicine* 154(12): 1365–70.

92. Thom, D. H., M. A. Hall, and L. G. Pawlson. 2004. Measuring patients' trust in physicians when assessing quality of care. *Health Affairs* 23(4): 124–32.

93. Ambady, N., D. Laplante, T. Nguyen, R. Rosenthal, N. Chaumeton, and W. Levinson. 2002. Surgeons' tone of voice: A clue to malpractice history. *Surgery* 132(1): 5–9.

94. Stewart, M. A. 1984. What is a successful doctor-patient interview? A study of interactions and outcomes. *Social Science and Medicine* 19(2): 167–75.

95. Roter, D. L., et al. 1997. Communication patterns of primary care physicians. *JAMA* 277(4): 350–56.

96. Maynard, D., and P. Hudak. 2008. Small talk, high stakes: Interactional disattentiveness in the context of prosocial doctor-patient interaction. *Language in Society* 37(5): 661–68.

97. Coe, J., C. Adams, and B. Bonnett. Prevalence and nature of cost discussions during clinical appointments in companion animal practice. *Journal of the American Veterinary Medical Association* 234(11): 1418–24.

98.   Eliot, V. S. 2003. Doctors use new cues to get patient history. *American Medical News,* June 23.

99.   Barrier, P. A., J. T. Li, and N. M. Jensen. 2003. Two words to improve physician-patient communication: What else? *Mayo Clinic Proceedings* 78(2): 211–14.

100. Hall, J. A., D. L. Roter, and N. R. Katz, 1988. Meta-analysis of correlates of provider behaviour in medical encounters. *Medical Care* 26(7): 657–75.

101. Maister, D. *Do you really want relationships.* http://davidmaister.com/articles/2/80/.

102. Sobel, A. 2008. *What drives client loyalty?* http://www.eyesonsales.com/content/article/what_drives_client_loyalty/.

103. Maister, D. 1997. *How to give advice.* http://davidmaister.com/articles/2/26/.

104. Pashler, H., M. McDaniel, D. Rohrer, and R. Bjork, R. 2008. Learning styles: Concepts and evidence. *Psychological Science in the Public Interest* 9(3): 105–19.

105. Massa, L. J., and R. E. Mayer. 2006. Testing the ATI hypothesis: Should multimedia instruction accommodate verbalizer-visualizer cognitive style? *Learning and Individual Differences* 16(4): 321–35.

106. http://en.wikipedia.org/wiki/Kinesthetic_learning.

107. Jackson, C. 2001. It pays to listen: The importance of doctor-patient communication. *American Medical News,* May 21.

108. Shaw, J. R. 2005. Four core communication skills of highly effective practitioners. *Veterinary Clinics of North America, Small Animal* 36(2): 385–95.

109. Gagliano, M. 2010. *How to use silence.* http://perigeebooks.typepad.com/blog/2010/09/how-to-use-silence.html.

110. http://www.ehow.com/info_8454395_clinical-interviewing-techniques.html

111. Howard, F. M. *History-taking and interview techniques and the physician-patient relationship.* http://www.glowm.com/resources/glowm/cd/pages/v6/v6c072.html?SESSID=jmfu0eh548ij1 7b5d35fl9nap4#the.

112. Sandman, P. 1987. Risk communication: Facing public outrage. *U.S. Environmental Protection Agency Journal (*November): 21–22.

113. Covello, V. *Risk communication: Principles, tools, and techniques.* Global Health Technical Briefs. Baltimore: Center for Risk Communication.

114. Cornell, K., and M. Kopcha. 2007. Client centered dialogue and shared decision making. *Veterinary Clinics of North America* 37(1): 41.

115. Adam, C. L., and S. M. Kurtz. 2006. Building on existing models from human medical education to develop a communication curriculum in veterinary medicine. *Journal of Veterinary Medical Education* 33(1): 28–37.

116. Lue, T. W., D. P. Pantenburg, and P. M. Crawford. 2008. Impact of the owner-pet and client-veterinarian bond on the care that pets receive. *Journal of the American Veterinary Medical Association* 232(4): 531–40.

117. Bonvicini, K., and S. Abood. 2006. Communicating with the client: Enhancing compliance. *Proceedings from Hill's Global Symposium on Feline Care,* 35–43.

118. Shaw, J., and B. Boynton. 2006. Communicating with the client: Enhancing compliance. *Hills Symposium on Dermatology,* 46–48.

119.   Greto, V. 2003. Pet lovers pay a price to keep animals fit. *The News Journal,* August 3.

120.   Flaim, D. 2003. Weighing dollars vs. dogs: A good relationship with your pet's vet is worth paying for. *Newsday,* June 24.

121.   Makoul, G. 2001. Essential elements of communication in medical encounters: The Kalamazoo consensus. *Academic Medicine* 76(4): 390–93.

122.   Morris, D. H. *Sympathy and empathy: What's the difference?* http://ezinearticles.com/?Sympathy-and-Empathy:-Whats-the-Difference?&id=5403134.

123.   Batmanabane, V. 2008. Empathy: A vital attribute for doctors. *Indian Journal of Medical Ethics* 5(3), 128–29.

124.   Fortin, A. H. 2002. Communication skills to improve patient satisfaction and quality of care. *Ethnicity and Disease* 12(4): S3-58–61.

125.   Boyle, D., B. Dwinnell, and F. Platt 2005. Invite, listen and summarize: A patient-centered communication technique. *Academic Medicine* 80(1): 29–32.

126.   Kim, S. S., and S. Kaplowitz. 2004. The effects of physician empathy on patient satisfaction and compliance. *Evaluation and the Health Professions* 27(3): 237–51.

127.   Silverman, J., S. A. Kurtz, and J. Draper. 1999. *Skills for communicating with patients.* Abingdon, England: Radcliffe Medical Press.

128.   Suchman, A. L., K. Markakis, H. B. Beckman, and R. Frankel. 1997. A model of empathic communication in the medical interview. *JAMA* 277(8): 678–82.

129.   Levinson, W., R. Gorawara-Bhat, and J. Lamb. 2000. A study of patient clues and physician responses in primary care and surgical settings. *JAMA* 284(8): 1021–27.

130.   Platt, F. W. 1992. Empathy: Can it be taught? *Annals of Internal Medicine* 117(8): 700.

131.   Hardee, J. 2003. An overview of empathy. *Permanente Journal* 7(4): 51–54.

132.   Darwin, C. 1872. *The expression of the emotions in man and animals.* London: John Murray.

133.   Carson, C. 2007. Nonverbal communication. *Veterinary Clinics of North America* 37(1): 49–63.

134.   Mehrabian, A., and S. Ferris. 1967. Inference of attitudes from nonverbal communication in two channels. *Journal of Consulting Psychology* 31(3): 248–52.

135.   *Using body language.* http://changingminds.org/techniques/body/body_language.htm.

136.   Knapp, M. L., and J. A. Hall. 2007. *Nonverbal communication in human interaction.* 5th ed. Boston: Wadsworth.

137.   Floyd, K., and L. K. Guerrero. 2006. *Nonverbal communication in close relationships.* Mahwah, NJ: Erlbaum.

138.   Verdon, D. R. 2003. Euthanasia's moral stress: A high psychological price. *DVM Newsmagazine,* July 1.

139.   Albert, A., and K. Bulcroft. 1988. Pets, families, and the life course. *Journal of Marriage and the Family* 50(2): 543–52.

140.   Gage, M., and R. Holcomb. 1991. Couples' perception of stressfulness of death of the family pet. *Family Relations* 40(1): 103–5.

141.   Nogueira, B. L. J., C. L. Adams, B. N. Bonnett, J. R. Shaw, and C. S. Ribble. 2010. Use of the measure of patient-centered communication to analyze euthanasia discussions in companion animal practice. *Journal of the American Veterinary Medical Association* 237(11): 1275–87.

142.   Durkin, A. Loss of a companion animal: Understanding and helping the bereaved. *Journal of Psychosocial Nursing & Mental Health Services* 47(7): 26–31.

143.   Lagoni, L., C. Butler, and S. Hetts. 1994. *The human-animal bond and grief*. Philadelphia: W. B. Saunders.

144.   Kübler-Ross, E. 1969. *On death and dying*. New York: Routledge.

145.   Kübler-Ross, E. 2005. *On grief and grieving: Finding the meaning of grief through the five stages of loss*. New York: Simon & Schuster.

146.   Planchon, L., D. Templer, S. Stokes, and J. Keller. 2002. Death of a companion cat or dog and human bereavement: Psychosocial variables. *Society & Animals* 10(1): 93–105.

147.   Tannenbaum, J. 1995. *Veterinary ethics: Animal welfare, client relations, competition and collegiality*. 2nd ed. St. Louis, MO: Mosby.

148.   Rebuelto, M. 2008. Ethical dilemmas in euthanasia of small companion animals. *Open Ethics Journal* 2: 21–25.

149.   Rollin, B. E. 2006. Euthanasia and quality of life. *Journal of the American Veterinary Medical Association* 228(7): 1014–16.

150.   Cartledge, R. 2008. *Killing healthy animals, an ethical dilemma?* http://etalk.sgu.edu/contribute/pawsprint/documents/KillingHealthyAnimalsRachelCartledge.pdf.

151.   Durrance, D., and L. Lagoni. 2010. *Connecting with clients: Practical communication for 10 common situations*. 2nd ed. Lakewood, CO: AAHA Press.

152.   *The CAHPS Improvement Guide: Practical strategies for improving the patient care experience—Training to advance physicians' communication skills*. https://www.cahps.ahrq.gov/qiguide/content/interventions/Training2AdvanceSkills.aspx.

153.   http://en.wikipedia.org/wiki/Conversation.

154.   Ryder-Smith J. 1998. The secret of good conversation—Investing in success. *Health Manpower Management* 24(1): 38–39.

155.   http://occonline.occ.cccd.edu/online/klee/CommunicationsStyleInventory.pdf.

156.   http://www.au.af.mil/au/awc/awcgate/sba/comm_style.htm.

157.   http://www.adventureassoc.com/workshops/myers-briggs/mbti-communication.html.

158.   http://www.mobiusmodel.com/downloads/positive_futures.pdf.

159.   Arikha, N. 2007. *Passions and tempers: A history of the humours*. New York: Ecco Press.

160.   Myers, I. B. 1995. *Gifts differing: Understanding personality type*. Mountain View, CA: Consulting Psychologists Press.

161.   Kroeger, O., with J. Thuesen and H. Rutledge. 2002. *Type talk at work: How the 16 personality types determine your success on the job*. Oakland, CA: Tilden Press.

162.   Berens, L. V., S. A. Cooper, L. K. Ernst, C. R. Martin, S. Myers, D. Nardi, R. R. Pearman, M. Segal, and M. A. Smith. 2001. *Quick guide to the 16 personality types in organizations: Understanding personality differences in the workplace*. Huntington Beach, CA: Telos.

163.   Allen, J., and S. Brock. 2000. *Health care communication using personality type*. New York: Routledge.

164.   Tieger, P. D., and B. Barron-Tieger. 1998. *The art of speed reading people*. New York: Little, Brown.

165. Keirsey, D. 1998. *Please understand me II.* Del Mar, CA: Prometheus Nemesis.

166. Brinkman, R., and R. Kirschner. 1994. *Dealing with people you can't stand.* New York: McGraw-Hill.

167. Reid, R. H., and D. W. Merrill. 1981. *Personal styles and effective performance.* Radnor, PA: Chilton.

168. Howard, P., and J. Howard. 2001. *The owner's manual for personality at work.* Austin, TX: Bard Press.

169. http://en.wikipedia.org/wiki/Keirsey_Temperament_Sorter.

170. Al-Jowaiser, M. M. 2004. Personality types and patient management in family practice. Paper presented at APT-XV, the 15th Biennial International Conference of the Association for Psychological Type, Toronto, Ontario, Canada.

171. Moutafi, J., A. Furnham, and J Crump. 2003. Demographic and personality predictors of intelligence: A study using the NEO Personality Inventory and the Myers-Briggs Type Indicator. *European Journal of Personality* 17(1): 79–94.

172. Kolb, D. A. 1984. *Experiential learning: Experience as the source of learning and development.* Englewood Cliffs, NJ: Prentice Hall.

173. Johnson, S., M. Gill, C. Grenier, and J. Taboada. 2009. A descriptive analysis of personality and gender at the Louisiana State University School of Veterinary Medicine. *Journal of Veterinary Medical Education* 36(3): 284–90.

174. Broida, J., L. Tingley, R. Kimball, and J. Miele. 1993. Personality differences between pro- and anti-vivisectionists. *Society and Animals* 1(2): 129–44.

175. Kimbal, R., and J. P. Broida. 1991. Psychological profiles of students for and against vivisection using the Myers-Briggs Type Indicator. *Humane Innovations and Alternatives* 5: 232–35.

176. Decety, J., C. Y. Yang, and Y. Cheng. 2010. Physicians down-regulate their pain empathy response: An event-related brain potential study. *Neuroimage* 50(4): 1676–82.

177. Chambers, R. 1993. Avoiding burnout in general practice. *British Journal of General Practice* 43(376): 442–43.

178. Hart, A. 1984. *Coping with depression in the ministry and other helping professions.* Lubbock, TX: Word.

179. Helpguide.org. *Preventing burnout: Signs, symptoms, causes and coping strategies.* www.helpguide.org/mental/burnout_signs_symptoms.htm.

180. Miller, L. 2004. JAVMA news: Managing stress and avoiding burnout. *Journal of the American Veterinary Medical Association* 225(4): ???.

181. Simonds, S. *Eleven simple ways to avoid burnout.* http://www.lifehack.org/articles/lifehack/11-simple-ways-to-avoid-burnout.html#.

182. Lloyd, J. W., and D. A. Walsh. 2002. Template for a recommended curriculum in "Veterinary Professional Development and Career Success." *Journal of Veterinary Medical Education* 29(2): 84–93.

183. Zeckhausen, W. 2002. Eight ideas for managing stress and extinguishing burnout. *Family Practice Management* 9(4): 35–38.

184.   Burns, G. A., K. L. Ruby, R. M. DeBowes, S. J. Seaman, and J. K. Brannan. 2006. Teaching non-technical (professional) competence in a veterinary school curriculum. *Journal of Veterinary Medical Education* 33(2): 301–8.

185.   Brazeau, C. M., R. Schroeder, S. Rovi, and L. Boyd. 2010. Relationships between medical student burnout, empathy, and professionalism climate. *Academic Medicine* 85(10): S33–36.

186.   Eliason, B. C., C. Guse, and M. S. Gottlieb. 2000. Personal values of family physicians, practice satisfaction, and service to the underserved. *Archives of Family Medicine* 9: 228–32.

187.   Lewis, J. M., F. D. Barnhart, B. L. Howard, D. I. Carson, and E. P. Nace. Work satisfaction in the lives of physicians. *Texas Medicine* 89(2): 54–61.

188.   Matheny, G. L. 2008. Money not key to happiness, survey finds. *Physician Executive* 34(6): 14–15.

189.   Quill, T. E., and P. R. Williamson. 1990. Healthy approaches to physician stress. *Archives of Internal Medicine* 150(9): 1857–61.

190.   Huggard, P. K., and E. J. Huggard. 2008. When the caring gets tough: Compassion fatigue and veterinary care. *VetScript*, May.

Resources

The Art of Speed Reading People, Paul D. Tieger and Barbara Barron-Tieger, 1998

Client Satisfaction Pays, Carin A. Smith, 2009

Communicating with Today's Patient, Joanne Desmond and Lanny R. Copeland, 2000

Communication High Wire, Dianne Saphiere and Barbara Mikk, 2005

Dealing with People You Can't Stand, Rick Brinkman and Rick Kirschner, 1994

Doctors Talking with Patients/Patients Talking with Doctors, Debra Roter and Judith Hall, 2006

Effective Client Communication in Veterinary Practice, special issue of *Veterinary Clinics of North America,* 37(1)

Five Steps to Professional Presence, Susan Bixler and Lisa Dugan, 2001

Gifts Differing, Isabel Briggs Myers, 1995

Health Care Communication Using Personality Type, Judy Allen and Susan Brock, 2000

How to Talk So People Will Listen, Steve Brown, 2005

It's Not the Dogs, It's the People, Nicole Wilde, 2003

The Leader Within, Human Synergistics International, 1999

Leveraging Your Communication Style, John Jackson and Lorraine Bosse-Smith, 2008

Please Understand Me II, David Keirsey, 1998

Type Talk at Work, Otto Kroeger with Janet Thuesen and H. Rutledge, 2002

Verbal Judo, Gerry Thompson and Jerry Jenkins, 2004

Index

A

Abstract information, 66

Acceptance, 39, 50

Advisor, 33–34

    client and, dynamic of, 31–32

    communication with, 31–33

AHA. *See* American Animal Hospital Association (AAHA)

Alternatives, 112

Ambady, Nalini, 27

American Animal Hospital Association (AAHA), 9, 11, 53

Anger, 50

Apathetic clients, Hawk as, 76

Architects. *See* Dreamer

Attachment, levels of, 47–48

Attentive body language, 43–44

Attire for veterinarian, 22–23

Auditory learners, 34

B

Bargaining, 50

Body language

    attentive, 43–44

    bored, 43–44

    disinterested, 43–44

    dominant, 44

Bored body language, 43–44

Brick wall, Dog as, 85–86

Burnout, communication for combating, 157–161

Burnout inventory, 167–168

C

Career, improved success of, 12

Career advancement opportunities, reduced, 158–159

Career and life, lack of balance in, 159

Champions. *See* Energizer

Client

    base for, increased, 6–9

    conflict, reduction in, 3–4

    as consumers, 19

    doctor, attire preferred by, 22

needs of, 15–20

neglect, educating on, 16

retention of, increased, 5–6

Closed-ended question, 30

Closing the deal, 10

Cognitive style, 60–62

decision making process, 66–68

definition of, 65

determining, 65–68

of Dog, 62, 83–84

of Dreamer, 124

of Energizer, 124

of Engineer, 123

of Hawk, 61, 73–75

hobby suggestions based on, 169

information gathering, 65–66

of Kitten, 62, 93–94

of Owl, 62, 103–105

social and, combination of, 73–75, 83–84, 93–94, 103–105, 169

types of, 57

veterinary personality and, 124

via FALE system, 111–115

Communicating with Today's Patient, 11

Communication

with advisors, 31–33

benefits of improved client, 3–12

burnout, for combating, 157–161

career, improved success of, 12

client base, increased, 6–9

client conflict, reduction in, 3–4

compensation, increase in, 11

compliance, improved, 9–11

with experts, 31–33

job satisfaction, for combating, 157–161

law suit, reduction in risk of, 4–5

retention of client, increased, 5–6

risk, 36–37

successful, defined, 18

work environment, improved, 11–12

Communication Assessment Tool, 55

Compensation, increase in, 11

Compliance, 9–11

empathy, 39–40

Composers. *See* Dreamer

Conflict, 3–4, 159

Connecting with Clients: Practical Communication for 10 Common Situations, Second Edition, 53

Consumers, client as, 19

Conversation style. *See also* Personality

with Dog, 145–146, 148–149, 148–150

with Hawk, 70, 145–148

importance of, 55

with Kitten, 146–147, 150–153

with Owl, 147–148, 153–155

quicksand, 145–155

of veterinarian, 117–122

Cost:benefit ratio, 10

CRAFT (Compliance = Recommendation + Acceptance + Follow Through), 9

Crafters. *See* Dreamer

Culture, 12

D

Darwin, Charles, 43

Data-driven information, 65–66

Deal, closing the, 10

Death, 52–53

Decision making process, 66–68

    empathetic, 67–68

    intelligent, 68

    logical, 67, 68

Denial, 50

Depression, 50

Detailed information, 65

Diagnostic options, 31–33

Difficult clients, handling of

    Dog, 82–83

    Hawk, 72–73

    Kitten, 93

Discoverers. *See* Energizer

Disinterested body language, 43–44

Distractions, 43, 44

Dog

    as brick wall, 85–86

    cognitive style of, 62, 83–84

    conversation style of, 80, 145–146, 148–153

    difficult clients, handling of, 82–83

    Dreamer, 84

    driving force of, 79

    emergencies, handling of, 81

    Energizer, 83–84

    Engineer, 84

    euthanasia of, 82

    financial costs of, 82

    grief of, 82

    information gathering for, 80

    Kitten and, truth about, 97–98

    Leader, 83

    medical problems, handling of serious, 81

    motto of, 79–80

    overview of, 79–81

    as parent, 84–85

    as rescuer, 86–87

    social style of, 83–84

    veterinary personality of, 128–132

Dominant body language, 44

Dominate vocal tones, 29

Dreamer

    cognitive styles of, 124

    Dog, 84, 131–132

    Hawk, 74–75, 127–128

    Kitten, 94, 135–136

    Owl, 104–105

    social style of, 60

E

Emergencies, handling of

    Dog, 81

    Hawk, 71

    Kitten, 92

    Owl, 102

Empathetic decision making, 67–68

Empathy, 37–42, 112

    compliance and, 39–40

    financial costs and, 40–41

    importance of, 41–42

End-of-life discussions, 47

Energizer

    cognitive styles of, 124

    Dog, 83–84, 129–130

    Hawk, 73, 126

    Kitten, 93, 134

    Owl, 104

    social style of, 60

Engineer

    Dog, 84, 130–131

    Hawk, 74, 127

    Kitten, 94, 134–135

    Owl, 104

    social style of, 59

Environment at work , improved, 11–12

Euthanasia, 48–53

    challenges encountered in, 48–49

    Dog, handling of, 82

    expected, 49–50

    Hawk, handling of, 72

    impulsive, 50–52

    Kitten, handling of, 92–93

    Owl, handling of, 103

    types of, 48

    unexpected (death), 52–53

Examination

    mental preparation for, 23

    physical, 31

    problem-oriented, 36–37

    purpose of, 29–30

Excessive workload, 158

Expected euthanasia, 49–50

Expert guide, 32

Experts, communication with, 31–33

Explorers. *See* Energizer

Expressions of the Emotions of Man and Animals, The (Darwin), 43

Ezekiel, 55

F

Facebook, 8

Fact-based information, 65–66

Facts, 112

    FALE system

    case studies on, 112–115

    cognitive style via, 111–115

    using, process for, 112–115

Fatigue, 44

Feelings, positive, 19

Field marshals, 59

Financial costs

    Dog, 82

    empathy for, 40–41

    Hawk, 71

    Kitten, 92

    Owl, 102–103

First impression, 27–28

Forbes, 8

Friendly talk, 29

G

Goals. *See* Personality

Grief

    communication during period of (*See* Euthanasia)

    Dog, handling of, 82

    Hawk, handling of, 72

    Kitten, handling of, 92–93

    Owl, handling of, 103

    stages of, 50

H

Happiness. *See* Personality

Harvard Business School, 31

Hawk

    as apathetic clients, 76

    cognitive style of, 61, 73–75

    conversation style of, 70, 145–151, 153

    difficult clients, handling of, 72–73

    driving force of, 69

    emergencies, handling, 71

    Energizer, 73

    Engineer, 74

    euthanasia of, 72

    financial costs of, 71

    grief of, 72

    Leader, 73

    medical problems, handling serious, 71

    motto of, 69–70

    overview of, 69–70

    social style of, 73–75

    as Spartans, 75–76

    veterinary personality of, 124–128

    victim's as, 76–77

Healers. *See* Dreamer

Hippocrates, 55

Hobby suggestions based on cognitive style, 169

Holloway, Pam, 24

I

Impulsive euthanasia, 50–52

Information

    abstract, 66

data-driven, 65–66

detailed, 65

for Dog, 80

explanation of, 17

fact-based, 65–66

gathering of, 65–66, 80, 90, 100

intuitive, 66

for Kitten, 90

for Owl, 100

specific, 65

up front presentation of, 17

variety of forms of, 18

Innate aspects of personality, 60

Inquiry, 29–33

advisor, role as, 31–34

closed-ended question, 30

diagnostic options, 31–33

experts, methods for communication with, 31–33

listening skills, 35

open-ended question, 30

physical exam, 31

purpose of examination, 29–30

resources, availability of, 34–35

silence, importance of, 35–36

treatment options, 31–33

Intelligent decision making, 68

Intuitive information, 66

J

JAVMA, 5

Job satisfaction, communication for combating, 157–161

K

Keirsey Temperament Sorter, 55

Kitten

cognitive style of, 62, 93–94

conversation style of, 90, 146–153, 155

difficult clients, handling of, 93

Dog and, truth about, 97–98

Dreamer, 94

driving force of, 89

emergencies, handling of, 92

Energizer, 93

Engineer, 94

euthanasia of, 92–93

financial costs of, 92

grief of, 92–93

information gathering for, 90

as know-it-all, 94–95

Leader, 93

medical problems, handling of serious, 91–92

motto of, 90

overview of, 89–91

social style of, 93–94

as storyteller, 96–97

veterinary personality of, 132–136

as wonderers, 95–96

Know-it-all, Kitten as, 94–95

L

Language barriers, overcoming, 18

Law suit, reduction in risk of, 4–5

Leader

cognitive styles of, 123

Dog, 83

Hawk, 73

Kitten, 93, 133

Owl, 103–104

social style of, 59

veterinary personality of, 125–126, 129

Leadership, poor, 159

Learners

auditory, 34

visual, 34

Lens of Understanding, 55

Leveraging Your Communication Style, 10

Life and career, lack of balance in, 159

Likeability, 23–25

Likeability Assessment, 25

Likeability Factor: How to Boost Your L-Factor and Achieve Your Life's Dreams, The (Sanders), 24

Likeability Quotient, 24

Listening skills, 35

Litigator, Owl as, 106–107

Logic, 112

Logical decision making, 67, 68

M

Maister, David, 31

Medical problems, handling of serious

Dog, 81

Hawk, 71

Kitten, 91–92

Owl, 101–102

prioritizing, 18–19

Medical terminology, use of, 18

Mental attitude, positive, 24

Mental preparation for examination, 23

Money talk, 10

Motivators. *See* Energizer

Motto

of Dog, 79–80

Hawk, 69–70

of Kitten, 90

of Owl, 100

Myers-Briggs Type Indicator, 55

N

Needs of client, 15–20

positive experience at clinic, 19–20

resolution of pet's problem, 16–19

respect for relationship with pet, 15–16

understanding of pet's problem, 16–19

Neglect, educating client on, 16

Nonjudgmental nature, 24

Nonverbal communication, defined, 21. *See also* Verbal and nonverbal communication during OFFICE call

O

OFFICE call. See Verbal and nonverbal communication during OFFICE call

Open-ended question, 30

Openness, 24

Outside exam room, 22–27

    likeability, 23–24

    mental preparation, 23

    physical preparation, 22–23

    self-image, 25–27

Owl

    cognitive style of, 62, 103–105

    conversation style of, 100, 147–155

    difficult clients, handling of, 103

    as doubting Thomas, 105–106

    Dreamer, 104–105, 140–141

    driving force of, 99

    emergencies, handling of, 102

    Energizer, 104, 138–139

    Engineer, 104, 139–140

    euthanasia of, 103

financial costs of, 102–103

grief of, 103

information gathering for, 100

Leader, 103–104, 137–138

as litigator, 106–107

medical problems, handling of serious, 101–102

motto of, 100

overview of, 99–101

as professor, 105–106

social styles of, 103–105

veterinary personality of, 136–141

as worrier, 107–108

P

Paraphrasing, 35

Parent, Dog as, 84–85

Pareto principle, 5

Perception, 36

Performers. *See* Energizer

Personal control, lack of, 158

Personal recommendation, 8

Personality. See also Veterinary personality

    assessment of, 118–122, 163–166

    innate aspects of, 60

    preferences of, 60

Perspectives of others, 25

Physical exam, 31

Physical preparation for examination, 22–23

Plato, 55

Positive experience at clinic, 19–20

Positive feelings, 19

Preferences of personality, 60

Problem-oriented exams, 36–37

Professor, Owl as, 105–106

Promoters. See Energizer

Purpose of examination, 29–30

Q

Questions

closed-ended, 30

open-ended, 30

Quicksand conversation, 145–155

Quixote, Don, 157

R

"Real" words, 18

Recognition, lack of, 158

Reflection, 35

Reid and Merrill's social styles, 55

Repeated movements, 44

Repetition, 35

Rescue group, 51, 87

Rescuer, Dog as, 86–87

Resolution of pet's problem, 16–19

Resources, availability of, 34–35

Respect for relationship with pet, 15–16

Retention of client, increased, 5–6

Risk communication, 36–37

S

Sanders, Tim, 24

Sandman, Peter, 36–37

Security, 25

Self-assessment of veterinarian, 117–122

Self-image, 25–27

"Seven Components of Likeability" (Holloway), 24

Silence, importance of, 35–36

Small talk, 29

Social style, 58–60

cognitive and, combination of, 73–75, 83–84, 93–94, 103–105, 169

of Dog, 83–84

of Dreamer, 60

of Energizer, 60

of Engineer, 59

Hawk, 73–75

hobby suggestions based on, 169

of Kitten, 93–94

of Leader, 59

of Owl, 103–105

Reid and Merrill's, 55

types of, 57

veterinary personality and, 124

Society for Prevention of Cruelty to Animals, 51

Spartans, 75–76

Specific information, 65

Status quo, 60

Stirring the pot, 60

Storyteller, Kitten as, 96–97

Successful communication, defined, 18

Supervisors, 59

Sympathy, 41–42

T

Tactile learners, 34–35

Teachers, 59

Temperaments, 60–61

Treatment options, 31–33

Twitter, 8

U

Understanding of pet's problem, 16–19

Unexpected euthanasia, 52–53

V

Verbal and nonverbal communication during OFFICE call, 21–45

empathy, 37–42

first impression, 27–28

friendly talk, 29

inquiry, 29–33

outside exam room, 22–27

problem-oriented exams, 36–37

risk communication, 36–37

Verbal communication, defined, 21. *See also* Verbal and nonverbal communication during OFFICE call

Verbal Judo: The Gentle Art of Persuasion, 4

Veterinarian

attire preferred by client, 22–23

conversation style of, 117–122

personality assessment of, 118–122

self-assessment of, 117–122

Veterinary Economics, 8, 9

Veterinary Medical Board, 5

Veterinary personality

cognitive style and, 124

Dogs, 128–132

field guide to types of, 123–144

Hawk, 124–128

Kitten, 132–136

Owl, 136–141

social style and, 124

U.S. norms, comparison with, 141–143

Victim's, Hawk as, 76–77

Videotaping, 28

Visual learners, 34

Vocal tones, 29

dominate, 29

warm, 29

Vulnerability, 25

W

Wall Street Journal (WSJ), 6–7, 16

Warm vocal tones, 29

Wonderers, Kitten as, 95–96

"Word-of-mouth" online reviews, 8

Work environment, improved, 11–12

Workload, excessive, 158

Worldviews. *See* Personality

Worrier, Owl as, 107–108

Y

Yellow Pages, 8

Yelp, 8

About the Author

Jon Klingborg, DVM, has published more than 250 newspaper articles, has coauthored a chapter in *Vet Clinics of North America,* has appeared on radio and television discussing veterinary issues and in print media around the world, was the youngest president in the history of the California Veterinary Medical Association, has served on committees of the American Veterinary Medical Association and the California Veterinary Medical Board, and has spoken nationally and internationally on animal welfare issues. Dr. Klingborg was awarded the honorary title of Distinguished Practitioner (DPNAP) by the National Academies of Practice in 2006.

Over the past 19 years, Klingborg has been a veterinary associate and an owner, practiced in rural and urban environments, has worked in small two-doctor and large multidoctor multilocation practices, and has been an exclusive practitioner of both mixed- and small-animal veterinary medicine. In each setting, he has used the power of communication to quickly build a loyal client base and provide high-quality medicine.

Dr. Klingborg earned undergraduate degrees in rhetoric and zoology (1987) and his doctorate in veterinary medicine (1992) from the University of California at Davis. For more than a decade, he also served as guest faculty at his alma mater and shared with veterinary students how communication makes practice more rewarding for both client and veterinarian.